I0493451

"ARABIC LANGUAGE LEARNING BY MEDICAL & PARAMEDICAL STAFF"

'SUPPLEMENT: COMMON USE ARABIC'.

PROFESSOR (DR.) ANIL K. SAHNI
B.Sc., M.B.B.S., M.S., F.I.C.S., Advanced D.H.A
SURGEON, MEDICAL TEACHER,
UROLOGIST, ENDOSCOPIST,
LITHOTRIPSY SPECIALIST.
Addresss: A-1/F-1 Block-A Dilshad Garden
Delhi-110095 India
Mobile : 09873083100
E-mail : dranil_sahni@yahoo.co.in
dranil_sahni@hotmail.com
dranilksahni@gmail.com
LIFE MEMBER :
AUSTRIAN MEDICAL SOCIETY
THE ASSOCIATION OF SURGEONS OF INDIA
DELHI UROLOGICAL SOCIETY
ASSOCIATION OF MINIMAL ACCESS SURGEONS OF INDIA
INDIAN ASSOCIATION OF GASTRO-INTESTINAL
ENDOSURGEONS
MEDICAL COUNCIL OF INDIA REG.No.:
3599(06.01.2005) / 27417(30.05.1983)U.P

PROFESSOR (DR.) ANIL K. SAHNI
B.Sc., M.B.B.S., M.S., F.I.C.S., Advanced D.H.A

PREFACE

The Necessity, Of A Text Of Arabic Language Learning,
By Non Arabic Speaking Medical And Paramedical Staff,
For Dealing Arabic Speaking Persons, Is An Important
Need, For All Times.

The Present Text, Comprises The Arabic
Translation Of Various Relevant Leading Questions,
Commands, Requests, Suggestions, Advises And Their
Expected Responses, Required By, Medical & Paramedical
Personnels, For Conducting Dealing With Arabic Speaking
Persons, In Completing Various Necessary Official
Formalities, Simultaneously Satisfying, The Necessary
Needs, In Regards To Clinical Acumen Of A Clinician,
With No Knowledge Of Arabic Language, By Offering,
Arabic Version/ Translation Of The Expected Conversation,
Needed To Reach At A Particular Diagnosis, By Age Old
Clinical Art Of History Taking, Clinical Examination,
Required Possible Investigations, To Conclude A Clinical
Diagnosis, And Then The Necessary Discussion For
Subsequent Treatment.

For The Validity Of The Present Text,
In An Attempt To Faciliate Communication, With The
Complete Arabic Population, Varying Expressions (
Classical, Colloquial, Masculine, Feminine, Singular,
Plural, Noun, Verbs, Adjective) For Conveying Almost
Same (Working Meaning) Has Been Included, To Provide
Reader, Availability Of A Choice, Modifying, As Deemed
Fit, By Personal Experiences, In Day To Day Practice.

In Process Consideration By, 'WHO', 'UN', "RED CROSS', 'RED CRESCENT', 'ICRC' & Other Authorities, The Book,"Arabic Language Learning by Medical & Paramedical Staff", Published, 2003, By Verification From, 'Government Of India', 'Office Of The Registrar Of News Papers For India', 'Ministry Of Information & Broadcasting', With Reprints.
In Reprint: 2009, "Supplement: Common Use Arabic" Additional About (50) Pages, Necessary For Immediate Day To Day Needs,Were Added.

In View Of Non-Availablity Of Such 'Study-Material', The Text, Is An Important Urgent Need For The Persons Going To, From These Countries. Several Copies Are In Use, At National & International Levels & In Constant Need, Throughout. This Next Edition, In Present Form Is Being Attempted.

PROF. (DR.) ANIL K. SAHNI
M.S, F.I.C.S, Advanced D.H.A.
Surgeon, Medical Teacher

"With Best Wishes & Special Thanks,
For Study Material Resources, Formats Etc.
And Moral Support."

"Arabic Language Learning
By Medical & Paramedical Staff"
'Supplement: Common Use Arabic'.

UNITED NATIONS INFORMATION CENTRE
55 Lodi Estate, New Delhi - 110 003

May 3, 2010

Dr. Anil K. Sahni
A-1/9-1, Block A
Dilshad Garden
Delhi- 110 095

Dear Sir,

We are pleased to confirm that your book entitled 'Arabic Language Learning by Medical & Paramedical Staff' has been received in our library.

Thanks and best regards,

Yours sincerely,

Dr. R.K. Sharma
Librarian

Telephones : 24623439, 46532333 Fax : 24620293, 24628508
e-mail : unicnvdin@unicindia.org

Acknowledgement   Wednesday, 12 November, 2008 4:06 PM

From: "RK Sharma" <rsharma@unicanda.org>

To: drani_sahni@yahoo.co.in
    image001.jpg (3KB)

Dear Dr. Sahni,

Thank you very much for sending the book- Arabic language learning......

We will put your name in our mailing list for sending UNews (A monthly Newsletter) to your changed
address.

Thanks

Dr. R.K. Sharma
Librarian
United Nations Information Centre
55 Lodi Estate, New Delhi- 110 003
Tel: 91-11-46532238, Fax 91-11-24620293, 24628900
Mobile: 9811807799
www.unic.org.in

image001.jpg

"Arabic Language Learning
By Medical & Paramedical Staff"
'Supplement: Common Use Arabic'.

Fax: 24673730
E-mail: dpll@vsnl.net

DELHI PUBLIC LIBRARY
GOVT. OF INDIA ORG., MINISTRY OF TOURISM AND CULTURE
(DELIVERY OF BOOKS ACT DIVISION)

Near Main Market,
Sarojini Nagar,
New Delhi-110023

Ref. No. DBAD.../.../...

Mrs. ....
....
....

1 6 MAY 2005

Sir,

Subject: Acknowledgement of books

We hereby acknowledge with thanks the receipt of the following books under Rule 3 of the Delivery of Books (Public Libraries) Rule 1955 delivered under Delivery of the Books and Newspapers (Public Libraries) Act, 1954.

1. Arabic Language Learning   16.
2. "By Medical & Paramedical staff
   copies)   17.
3.   18.
4.   19.
5.   20.
6.   21.
7.   22.
8.   23.
9.   24.
10.   25.
11.   26.
12.   27.
13.   28.
14.   29.
15.   30.

Yours faithfully,

Assistant Library & Information Officer

PROFESSOR (DR.) ANIL K. SAHNI
B.Sc., M.B.B.S., M.S., F.I.C.S., Advanced D.H.A

Ph :- 23991297
Website: www.delhipubliclibrary.in
E-mail: dpl@dpl.gov.in

DELHI PUBLIC LIBRARY
GOVT. OF INDIA ORC-MINISTRY OF CULTURE
(DELIVERY OF BOOKS ACT DIVISION)

S.P.Mukherjee Marg,
Opp. Old Delhi Railway Station
Delhi – 110006

Ref.No.DPL/DBAD/ EX /208   Date: 28/6/10

Mr. Dr. Anil K. Sahni.
A-1/F-1 Block-A
Dilshad Garden,
Delhi - 110095

Sir,

We hereby acknowledgement with thanks the receipt of the following books under Rule 3 of the Delivery of Books (Public Libraries) Rule 1955 delivered under Delivery of the Books and Newspapers (Public Libraries) Act,1954.

Please note under the said Act copies have also to be supplied to:

1. The National Library, Belvedere, Kolkata- 700027.
2. The Connemara Public Library, Egmore, Chennai- 600008.
3. The State Central Library, Town Hall, Mumbai- 400023.

1. Arabic language learning   9.
2.   (one book)   10.
3.   11.
4.   12.
5.   13.
6.   14.
7.   15.
8.   16.

Yours faithfully

Assistant Library & Information Officer

8.

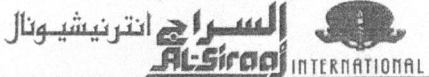

INTERNATIONAL

REF: ALS/MIH/09/10
DT.: 26.07.2009.

'TOWHOMSOEVER IT MAY CONCERN'

THIS IS TO CERTIFY THAT "TEXT," "ARABIC LANGUAGE LEARNING BY
MEDICAL AND PARAMEDICAL STAFF", BY DR. ANIL K. SAHNI. (M.S.F.I.C.S.
ADVANCED D.H.A.) , IS RECOMMENDED AND IS BEING USED BY SEVERAL
PERSONS, GOING ABROAD.

OUR ORGANISATION IS A GOVT. APPROVED RECRUITMENT AGENCY

WE WISH HIM ALL SUCCESS IN HIS BRIGHT FUTURE.

FOR AL-SIRAAJ INTERNATIONAL

(MEHMOOD ISMAIL HAMDULE)
MANAGING DIRECTOR

Office : 11-J (11th Floor), Gopala Tower,
25, Rajendra Place, New Delhi-110 008 (India)
Tel. : (+91-11) 25854786, 25824342
Fax : (+91-11) 25815786, 25787057
www.alsiraaj.com • e-mail : alsiraaj@vsnl.com

PROFESSOR (DR.) ANIL K. SAHNI
B.Sc., M.B.B.S., M.S., F.I.C.S., Advanced D.H.A

Dr. ANIL K. SAHNI
M.B.B.S., M.S., F.I.C.S.
SURGEON, UROLOGIST
LITHOTRIPSY SPECIALIST

LIFE MEMBER :
AUSTRIAN MEDICAL SOCIETY
THE ASSOCIATION OF SURGEONS OF INDIA

Phone : 22586072
22580837 (PP)
Mobile : 9873083100

A-1/F-1, Dilshad Garden,
Delhi-110095. INDIA

Date: Feb, 1998

To,
The Officer Incharge,
Publication Department,
WHO
IPEST
M. Gandhi Marg-2
Delhi.

Respected Sir,

With due regards, this is with reference to your letter dated 23 February, 1998. (Photocopy Attached), in response to the application (Photocopy Attached),

SUBJECT : "TEXT OF ARABIC LANGUAGE LEARNING, BY NON ARABIC CONVERSING MEDICAL & PARAMEDICAL STAFF, FOR DEALING ARABIC SPEAKING PERSONS"

Persuading the application to the, or, correspondance address of person concerned is requested.

With due thanks,

Sincerely yours,

(DR. ANIL K. SAHNI)

ENCLOSURES:
BIODATA OF THE AUTHOR (1)
TEXT 'SUBJECT DETAILS' (2)

"Arabic Language Learning
By Medical & Paramedical Staff"
'Supplement: Common Use Arabic'.

WORLD HEALTH ORGANIZATION
Regional Office for the Eastern Mediterranean
ORGANISATION MONDIALE DE LA SANTE
Bureau régional de la Méditerranée orientale

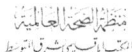

منظمة الصحة العالمية
المكتب الاقليمي لشرق المتوسط

W.AP.2.14

23 February, 1998

Dear Sir,

We refer to your undated letter regarding your request to obtain a sort of teaching material that allow non-Arabic speaking physicians to communicate with Arabic-speaking patients, etc. We are sorry not to be able to meet this request. WHO Arabic programme at EMRO is mainly concerned with converting WHO and other medical publications of interest to Arab member countries into Arabic for the sake of disseminating health and biomedical information in these countries.

Regards and thank you for writing to us.

M.J. Al-Khateeb
Head, WHO Arabic programme

Dr. Anil K. Sahni
A-1/F-1
Dilshad Garden,
Delhi,
India
c/o SEARO

P.O. BOX 1517 ALEXANDRIA (21511) EGYPT   D.P. 1517 ALEXANDRIE, EGYPTE   ص.ب. 1517 الإسكندرية (21511) جمهورية مصر العربية
TELEGR. UNISANTE, Alexandria   UNISANTE, Alexandrie   برقياً: يونيسانت ، الإسكندرية
☎ 48300/477/659 - 48.59240   TELEX 54028/54084 WHO UN تلكس: فاكس: FAX 4838916
E Mail/Courrier Electronic EMRO@WHO.SCI.EG   البريد الإلكتروني:

THROUGH HUMANITY TO PEACE

 Indian Red Cross Society

(CONSTITUTED UNDER ACT XV OF 1820)

Telegrams : "INDCROSS"
Telefax : 91-11-23717454
Phones : (PBX Lines) 23716441, 42, 43
Website : www.indianredcross.org
A-33015/01/13/DMC/library

Headquarters :
1, RED CROSS ROAD
NEW DELHI - 110 001

Date-08.03.2013

Dr. Anil Kumar Sahni
Surgeon
A-1/F1,Block A
Dilshad Garden,
Delhi-110095
INDIA
Telephone-09873083100 (M)
011-42331264 (R)

Subject-Acknowledgement of Arabic language learning by Medical & Paramedical staff (Supplement Common use Arabic)

Dear Sir,

We hereby acknowledge with thanks of above titles book useful for medical & paramedical staff users.

We wish all success in this bright future.

Yours Sincerely

(Hira Lal)
Librarian

12.

PART-(1)
"Arabic Language Learning By Medical & Paramedical Staff"

CONTENTS

Page

1. Particulars of the Patient 15

2. Numerals 17

3. Problems, Complains, Symptoms 20

4. Various Body Organs 24

5. Clinical History 30

6. Medical History, History of Previous Surgery,

   Family History, Social History, Occupational

   History 55

7. Clinical Examination 58

8. Investigations 61

9. Diagnosis : Disease 64

10. Treatment 65

11. Paramedical Staff 71

12. Medical Specialists...74

PART-(2)
'Supplement : Common Use Arabic'

CONTENTS

Page

I. Useful Arabic Expressions
   (A) Introductory 77
   (B) Understanding Language 80
   (C) Official 82
   (D) Usful Phrases
       Useful Vocabulary 85

II. Useful Grammar 102

III. Time, Week Days, Months, Seasons 113
    Cardinal Points, Colours,
    Human Relations Etc

Note:

The Varying Arabic Expressions Have Been
Differentiated By-
- COMA (,) For The Words Conveying
  Same Meaning,
- COLON (:) From English Expressions &
- SEMICOLON (;) Has Been Used To
  Differentiate In Between.

CHAPTER—1
Particulars of the Patient

Peace be Upon You : Assalam Alay Kum

In Reply : Wa Alay-Kum Assalam

Patient, Sick : Maridh, Mareeth, Pl. Mardha

Ambulance : Sayaarat-al-is-Aaf

Accompany (With) : You Raafiq, Rafaq, Yurafiq
(Ma, Wiya)

Attendant : Murafaq

Registration : Taqyid

Document : Wathiqa, Mustanid, Sened

File : Seff, Malaf

Prescription : Warga Elaaj, Wasfa

Bed Number : (Number) Raqem/Nimrae,
(Bed) Sareer/Firash

Visit : Ziyara, Pl. Ziyarat

Please, come here : (Please) Min Fathlak/Min
Fadhlek; Taal Hana (Come Here)
Colloquial : Fatth, Fadh Pl. Fadal, Fadhal; Taal Hena

Wait : Istandhar, Yastadhir V.
Colloquial : Istania, Stania

Please Sit Down : Tafadal Ejles (M), Tafadal
Ejlesi (F) Colloquial : Gaams

What Is Your Name : Shinu Asmak (M), Shinu
Asmik (F) Colloquial : Ismak

What Is Your Age : Kam Umrak (M), Kum Umrik (F)
Colloquial : Umr

Sex : Jins

Male : Dhikr, Thakar Pl. Dhukur

Female : Niswan, Nisa, Muannat, Harma Mara, Pl.
Harim,

Eunch : Khasi, Pl. Khisyan, Mukshi, Makhasi

Height : Ilu, Irtifa Colloquial : Tool

Tall : Tawil

Short : Qaseer, Qasir, Pl. Qisar

Dwarf : Kawam

Weight : Thaqil : Heavy, Wazn,

Obese : Samin

Thin : Nahif

Nationality : Jinsiya, Al-Jensiya

CHAPTER—2
Numerals

0 : Sifr

1 : Wahed

2 : Et-Nain, Zouz

3 : Ta-Laat

4 : Ar-Baa

5 : Khamsa

6 : Sitta

7 : Sab-Aa

8 : Tamanaya

9 : Tis-Aa

10 : Ash-Raa

11 : Eh-Daash

12 : At-Naash

13 : T'Lataash

14 : Ar-Bataash

15 : Khams-Taash

16 : Sitta-Sh

17 : Saba-Tash

18 : T' Man-Tash

19 : T'Ssa-Tash

20 : Esh-Reen

21 : Wahed Wa Esh-Reen

22 : Etnain Wa Esh-Reen, Zouz Wa Esh-Reen

23 : T'Laata Wa Esh-Reen

24 : Ar-Baa Wa Esh-Reen

25 : Khamsa Wa Esh-Reen

26 : Sitta Wa Esh-Reen

27 : Sab-Aa Wa Esh-Reen

28 : T'Manya Wa Esh-Reen

29 : Tis-Aa Wa Esh-Reen

30 : Talaateen

40 : Ar-Ba-Een

50 : Khamseen

60 : Sitteen

70 : Sab-Een

80 : T'Maneen

90 : T'Ss-Een

100 : Meeya

200 : Meetain : Etnain Meeya :Zouz Meeya

1000 : Alf

2000 : Alfain, Etnain Alf : Zouz Alf

1,000,000 : Malyoun

2,000,000 : Malyounain : Etnain "Alf" :
Zouz "Alf" (Hundreds)
3,000,000 : Talat Malayeen

Quarter : Rooba : Fourth Part : Rub, Pl. Arba,

Half : Nesf, Nuss, Nusf

And : Wa, Addition : Zum

No, Less, Sustraction : Illa, Aqall, Naqis, Tarh

"Arabic Numerals"
0 : Sifr ; ٠
1 : Wahed ; ١
2 : Et-Nain, Zouz ; ٢
3 : Ta-Laat ; ٣
4 : Ar-Baa ; ٤
5 : Khamsa ; ٥
6 : Sitta ; ٦
7 : Sab-Aa ; ٧
8 : Tamanaya ; ٨
9 : Tis-Aa ; ٩
10 : Ash-Raa ; ١٠

CHAPTER—3
Problems, Complains, Symptoms

What Is Your : Shenu (You), Kaeff (What),

Complain Matha, (Is) Fee Mushkilaat
Colloquial : Kaeff/Matha Mushkila, Fee Mushkila,
Kaeff/Matha

Please Tell, Talk, Say : Fadhal, Fadal, Pl. Fatth, Fadh,
Kalam (Tell, Talk, Say)

Complain : Ishtaka, Yashteki

Problem : Mesela, Masayil Pl.

Problematical : Mushkil

Duration : Min Kam Youm
Colloquial : Kam Youm,
Kam Waqt, Geedaas Waqt

Minute : Daqeeqa, Digheegha

Hour : Saa

Day : Youm

Week : Esboo

Month : Shahar

Year : Sana

Since Birth : Min Walada Colloquial : Mama, Umm,
Walida; Kaalam

Hereditary : Irthi, Warathi

Symptom : Alama

Pain : Thuja, Huja, Alam, Waja

Colic : Maksha

Abdominal Colic : Batni Tilwi

Severe : Shadeed

Less : Aaqal

Continuous : Daiman, Kull Waqt

Often : Kathir Marrat, Wajid

Sometimes : Badh Waqt, Waqti, Fourie

Lump, Mass, Tumour, Swelling : Khees, Keff

Warm : Wurum, Dumla, Tulu

Size : Kubr, Hazm

Small : Saghir, Shoya

Large : Kabeer Colloquial : Halba

Soft : Leyyin

Hard : Qawi

Stony : Muhajjar, Hajari

Increase : Eezeed, Zaada, Izdiyad, Ziyada

Swell : V. Waram, Yoram

Slow : Batee, Thaqil

Fast : Saree

Suddenly : Fuzatan, Defatan

Hematoma : Nezf Dhakhil (Haemorrage)

Abscess : Habba, Khorraj

Lympth Node : Tadakum Gudad Allemf
Enlargement

Fever, Pyrexia : Harara, Duration
Continuous, Intermittent

Associated (With) : Ma, Wiya
Chills and Rigor (Cold) : Barid,
Evening Rise : Saad Yasad Mesa (Evening)
Temperature Harara (Temperature)

Night Sweats : Mushkila Laila Araq

Pattern : Namuna, Pl. Namayin

Hyperpyrexia : Suhuna Zaida

Injury, Trauma : Dharar, Isaba, Madharra,Dharba

Blow : Habb, Yahibb, Dharba

Hit : N. Sawab

Accident : Musiba, Musayib

Accidentally : Bita Saduf

Traffic : Rayih Jai (Passing To And Fro)

Transportation : Naqliya

Laceration : Tamzig

Bruise : Damdama, Rusus, Balgusha

Stab : Taan, Yatan

Arms : Islah, Asliha

Gun (Rifle) : Tufka, Pl. Tufek

Machine Gun : Rash shash, Mitralyoz

Shooting (Firing) : Rami

Small Bullets : Sechem

Cannon Ball : Gulla, Pl. Gulel

Cannon : Top, Atwap, Medfa, Pl.Madafi

Blow : Yanfukh

Explosion : Infijar

Explode : Infejer

Mine : Lughm, Pl. Algham, (In War)

CHAPTER—4
Various Body Organs

Body : Jised, Jasad, Beden

Organ part : Adhu, Pl. Adha

Head : Raaass, Pl. Ruus

Skull : El-Gum-Goha, Zum Zuma

Skull Cap : Araqchin

Brain : Mukh, Dimagh

Forehead : Gassa, Jabin

Scalp : Zild, Zilud ; (Skull)

Skull : Shaar Arras

Hair : Shara, Shaar, Pl. Shar

Eye (S) : Ain (S), Pl. Ayoun

Eye Lid : El-Gif-Ne, Jifn, Pl. Jifun

Eye Lashes : El-Roo-Moosh

Eye Brow : Hajib, Hawajib

Lacrimal Gland : G. Addamaa

Ear (S) : Uthun (S), Athaan (Pl.),Idhn, Pl. Adhan

Nose : Khashim, Khashm

Nostril : Mankhara, Pl. Manakhir

Nasal Sinuses : Juyoub Anfiya

Tongue : Lissan, Pl. Elsina

Throat : Henjara

Tonsils : Ael Liwaezz

Adenoids : Rudhedat

Larynx : Haak

Pharynx : Bulum

Colloquial : Malaq

Thyroid Gland : G. Darakiya

Salivary Gland : G. Alloab

Parotid Gland : Gudda Nokafiya

Face : Wajah, Pl. Wujuh

Cheek : Khaad, Pl. Khudud

Jaw : El-Fak, Fekk, Fech

Chin : Id-Da-Ne, Dhuqn, Lehya

Mouth : Fam, Fah Colloquial :Halaq, Pl. Huluq

Lip : Shiffa, Shifa, Pl. Shifaf

Moustache : Shawarib

Beard : Lehya, Pl. Liha, Zaken

Teeth : Asnan, Sinn, Pl. Isnan

Gums : Roqba, Ruqba

Neck : El-lis-sa

Chest : Sadr, Fuwad

Ribs : Duluu

Heart : Qalb, Ghalb

Pericardium : Tam Up.

Heart Inner Part : Batn

Atrium : Uzeyn

Ventriculum : Buteyn

Aorta : Aorta

Diaphargm : Hizab-Hajiz, Assitara

Pleura : Pleura

Lung (S) : Ree-A, Ree-Ya, Riyaten

Breast : Saedy, Sadr, Pl. Sudur

Nipple : Memma

Abdomen : Bat-N

Umblicus, Navel : Surrah

Oesophagus : Merri

Liver : Kabda, Kebeb

Spleen : Tahal, Tadhyil, Tohal

Gall Bladder : Meraash, Marrara

Stomach : Maa-Ida, Mada

Duodenum : Ithny Ashar

Intestines : Masarin

Small Intestine : Ama Rakika

Large Intestine : Ama Galiba

Caecum : Musran Aawar

Ascending Colon : Colon Said

Appendix : Zaida, Tadhyil

Rectum : Mustakim

Anus : Sharaj

Loins : Janb

Kidney : Kil-Wa, Pl. Kilawi

Ureter : Halib

Bladder : Maesaenae, Mathana

Sex Organs : Udu, Attansul

Penis : Athakar, Algalem

Testicle : Khisia

Uterus : Rahim

Ovarium, Ovary, Ovum: Mibyab, Buwayda

Vagina : Mihbal

Vulva : Faraj

Front : Jabha

Back : Dahree, Dhahr, Pl. Dhuhur

Shoulder : Katif, Kitf, Pl. Aktaf, Atiq, Pl. Awatiq

Shoulder Blade : Deffa

Collar : Yakha, Pl. Yakhat, Towq

Axilla : Bat

Armpit : Tahtel, Bat

Arm : Dhiraa, The-Raa, Kitf, Pl. Aktaf, Dhra,

Pl.Vdhru,Ziraa

Elbow : Mirfaq, Aks

Wrist : Mi-Sam, Khasr

Hand (S) : Yad (S), Pl. Yadain, Edi, Pl.Edi, Id, Yed, Yedeya

Palm of Hand : Keff

Finger (S) : Saba (S), Pl. Asaaba, Usbu,Pl. Asabi, Subsabaya

Pelvis : Hawd, Id

Hip : Raedf, Warq, Warj

Leg (S) : Saagh (S), Pl. Seghaan, Rijl, Pl. Rijjul, Riyul

Foreleg : Rijl Qadamania

Hindleg : Rij Warania, Dual Rejlen Warania

Knee : Rok-Ba, Rukba, Pl. Rukub, Rukabh

Ankle : Kasabit Ae Rigl

Foot, Feet : Kadam (S), Akdaam (Pl.),Rijl, Pl. Rijjul, Pl. Riyul

Heel : Ka-Ab

Toe : Asbaa Ael Kadam, Usbuer Rizl, Pl. Asabi, Sub Er Rizl

Tarsus : Misht El Rizl

Limbs : Atraf

Nail : Dhafr, Pl. Adhafer, Adhafir, Zufur

Membrane : Ghasha

Skin : Jild, Jiled, Jilub

Blood Vessel : Damar, Pl. Damarat

Vein : Irk, Pl. Uruq

Artery : Shoryaen, Damar, Pl.Damarat

Nerve : Asab

Muscle : Adal, Adalat, Habra, Pl.Habr

Skeleton : Hekal

Bone : Aedaam, Adhm, Pl. Adham

Marrow : Mukhkh

Spine : Sansur

Vertebrae : Fakarat

Joint : Uqda, Pl. Uqad, Uqud,

Mafsal, Pl. Mafasil

Side : Janib, Yamil

Left : Yasaarak

Right : Yameenak

Unilateral, One Side : Wahed; Yamil, Janib

Two Side, Bilateral : Etnain, Zouz; Janib, Yamil

CHAPTER—5
Clinical History
Various Body Systems

Have Been Discussed As :

I. Anatomical Structures

II. Symtomatology

III. Common Diseases

System : Nidham, Tarz, Nasq, Tertib

I. *Central Nervous System*
Head Injury
Head : Raaans, Pl. Ruus; **Injury :** Dharar, Isaba, Madharra, Dharba; **Blow :** Habib, Yahibb, Dharba; **Hit :**N. Sawab.

Level of Conciousness Drowsy : Naiis

Unconciousness : Mayahiss

Commatose : Gairwayi

Orientation (Time,

Place, Person) ; Place : This

Place : N. Makan, Pl. Amakin,Mahall, Pl. Mahallat

Nausea : Gafayan, Laben Nefs

Nauseate : Yulaib

Vomitting : Ekdif, Kaei, Radda,Taqayya, Yazu, Yastafrigh,Yataqayya

Bleeding ENT : Nezf (Bleeding)

Ear : Uthun, Idhn, Pl. Athaan, Adhan

Nose : Khashim, Khashm

Mouth : Fam, Fah

Colloquial : Halaq, Pl.

Huluq : Throat

Convulsions : Khadda, Raasha

Neurological Deficit : Ghabat Ruhuh, Asab Ajz
Other Diseases

Head : Raans, Pl. Ruus; **Injury :** Dharar, Isaba,
Madharra, Dharba; **Blow :** Habib, Yahibb, Dharba;
Hit :N. Sawab.

Headache : Sudaa, Waja Ras

Throbbing : Khafaqan

Epilepsy : Assaraa

Rabies : Inkilab

Hydrophobia : Keleb

Parkinsonism : Arraash

Sciatica : Irkannisa

Hemi Plegia : Shalal, Shalal Nisfi

Ence Phalitis : Iltihab Almukh

Meningitis : Iltihab Assahaya

Neurology

Faculty Memory : Edh Dhakira

Neuralgia : Nawazil

Faculty of Sense : Hass

Sensation : Hassa, Ihsas

Numb : Mukhaddar

Sense Less, Unconcious,

Neurological Deficit : Ghabat Ruhuh, Asab Ajz

Palsy, Paralysis : Falij

Paralytic : Mafluj

Jerk : Hizza

Ataxic : Yatamyil

Flaccid : Markhi

Tremors : Arraasha

Gait : Meshi

Psychiatary

IQ: Intelligence : Kharij, Nisbat Addakaa
Quotient

Mentally Retarded : Daafakli, Aqlan, Awwaq,Yuawwiq

Intelligent : Thakey, Aqil, Fahim, Pl. Uqqal, Fahimin

Mental : Aqli

Mentally : Aqlan

Temperament : Akhlaq, Tabia

Good Tempered : Taayib-El-Akhlaq

Bad Tempered : Redi-El-Akhlaq

Tranquil : Hadi, Sakin

Tranquility : Hudu

Steady : Taabeit

Stability : Thabat

Agitated : Maqluq

Anger : Zal, Mughtadh

Irritable : Hadd El Mizaj, Mutawattir

Restless : Rahat Siz

Impulsive : Sari-Ette-Eththur

Nervous : Asabi

Nervousness : Asabiya

Sleep : N. Nom

33

Insomnia : Gelic Annown

Strain : Khal Khala

Faculty of Imagination : Takhayul

False Idea ; Delusion : Hallucination : Wahm

Visionary Unreal : Wahmi

Apparition : Khayal

Sane : Sahih-El-Aql

Insane : Majnun, Mukhabbal, Pl.

Majanin, Makhabil

Insanity : Junun, Khabal

Hypochondria : Soda

Melancholic : Sodawi

Maligneering : Mutamarid

II. *Opthalmology : Opthalmics*

Blind : Amya, Ama, Pl. Amyanin

Vision : Eyesight : Shoof, Basr

Refraction : Inkisar

Conjunctivitis ; : Iltihab
Inflammation

Tear : From Eye : Dema, Damaa, Pl. Duhu

Redness : Hamra

Sticky Eyes : Enitzabbit

Glaucoma : Mai Aswad

Squint, Strabismus : V. Ahwal, Alhawal

Spectacles : Mandhara, Pl. Mandharat,

Cataract:Manadhir

Sunglasses : Em-Rayaat

Surgery for Vision : Amaliyah – Shoof

III. *E.N.T. : Ear, Nose, Throat*

Sense of Hearing : Sem

Hear : Sema, Yisama

Colloquial : Isma

Deaf : Atrash, F.Tarsha, Pl. Tursh

Vertigo : Dukha

Vertige : Rasiydoor

Sense of Smell : Shemm

Perforate : Naqab, Yinqab, Yanqab

Discharge ; Nasal : Madda Min Almahbil

Discharge

Mucus : Mukhat

Cattarh : Zukam

Influenza : Influenza

Sneezing : Al Lattis

Mute : Bakkush

Faculty of Speech : Nutq

Whisper : Wash Washa

IV. *Endocrinology*

Thyroid : G. Darakiya
Goitre : Tumor Thyroid
Swelling In Front : Khees, Keef (Swelling);
Of Neck Moving With Jabha (Front) ; Roqba, Ruqba
Deglutition ; (Neck); Waqte Yakul,
Tahwil, Sherba (Deglutition);
Fithna, Tabdil Hea (During);
Mawqa, Makan Pl. Mawaqi,Amakin (Moving)

Tachycardia : (Increase) Akthar, Ezyed;
Hasab, Yahsab, Galb, Qalb (Heart Rate)
Affliction Nerves : Asabiya
Psychiatric Manifestations: Mushkila Hsasiya
Geographical : Joghrafi, Tawzi Variation,
Distribution (Distribution) : Ikhtilaf, Taghayyur
*Diabetes:***Mushkila Sukkar, Bowl Sukkari**
Polydypsoea : Kathir Alaatish, Akthar Ezyed
(Increase) Atash (Thirst)
Thirsty : Atshan
Poly phagia : Kathir Aljuu, Kathir Alakil.
Akthar Ezyed Ishtiha(Appetite) Ju (Hunger),
(Hungry) Joan, Pl. Joanin,Jowaa
Polyuria : Kathir Akthar, Ezyed Bol
Delayed Healing : (Delayed) Akhkhar,Mutaakhkhir,
Shafa, Shefa, Shifa (V.) (Healing)
Treatment
Oral Hypoglycaemic Agents : Haboob
Insulin
Duration : Min Kam Youm,
Colloquial : Kam Youm, Kam Waqt, Geedaas Waqt

V. *Respiratory System*

Respiratory Problem : Mushkila Tenefuss

History Suggestive of Tuberculosis : Daqq, Sull

Weight Loss : Aqal Wazn, Nagis Wazin

Appetite, Hunger : Aqal (Less), Ishtiha, Joanin,

Loss ; Nagis Shahiya

Evening : Rise : Temperature
: Mesa : Saad, Yasad, Harara

Night Sweats : Mushkila Lela Arq.

Cough : Kahha, Gahha, Gahh, Yaguhh

Secretion : Tefel, Yitfal : Nakhama

Expectoration

Dry Cough : No Secrtion

Productive Cough : Yagtaa

Amount : Quantity : Miblagh, Pl. Mabaligh Miqdar

Color : Rang, Lon, Pl. Alwan

Odor : Smell; Ishtemm, Yeshtemm

Foul Smell : Filthy; Wasikh

Haemoptysis : Sputum Blood; Yikuhdam

Cyanotic : Azrak

Dysnoea : Mushkila Tenefuss

Severity : Sarama

Mild : Nuss, Nesf

Moderate : Mutedil, Mutawassit

Severe : Excessive; Shadid

Tachypnoea : Akthar, Ezyed, Hasab, Yahsab, Tenefuss

Orthopnoea : Postural Dysnoea; Mushkila
Tenefuss : Khaffaf, Yukhaffif (Make Easy, Releive) :
(During) Ithna, Tabdil,Taghyir, Yughayer, Badaala
(Posture) Hea, Mawqa, Pl.Mawaqi, Makan, Pl. Amakin ;
(Sitting) Gaams,Yaqad, Jeles, Yizlas

Tachypnoea : Exertional Dysnoea ; Akthar,
Ezyed, Hasab, Yahsab,
Tenefuss Mushkila Tenefuss
Badein Shoghl, Riyadha

Gasp : Shehga

Wheezing Chest : Sodri Yizawi

**History Suggestive of Previous Treatment ;
Gabl, Sabiq, Qabal (Previous)** : Elaaj (Treatment)
:(Duration) Kam Youm, KamWaqt ; Geedas Waqt
Previous : Papers **Prescriptions**

Regarding Treatment : Gabl, Sabiq (Previous)
Qabal : Wasfa, Warga Elaaz (Treatment Papers)
Wain, Menain (Where)

Possible Glance : Mumkin; Lefta, Shoof

Treatment Compliance,

Adherence : Elaaz, Kull, Waqt, Youm; Confirm : Haqqaq,

Yuhaqqiq Colloquial : Mazboot

Treatment Where : Elaaz ; Wain, Menain

Hospital ; Mustashfa : Ismak (Name)

Residence : Bayat, Hoosh

Details Treatment ; Tablet,Capsule, Injection

Duration

Control After Complete Treatment Radiology

(X Ray Chest) Normal : Bedein Kullelaaz , Surra Sadr : Aadii, Taebi

Social History :

Smoker :

Disease in the Family : Usra

Neighbour : Jarr, Jirain

Neighbourhood : Mahalla

Occupational Respiratory Diseases
(Other Diseases)

Tuberculosis : Daqq, Dharan, Sull

Pleurisy : Dhat El Jenb

Pneumonia : Dhat Er Riya, Marad Arragig Iltihaab Sadr

Allergic Respiratory : Bronchial Asthma, Asthma;

Diseases Fadda, Azma, Rabuu

Lung Tumor : Khinzirah, Sarataan Sadr

VI. *Cardiovascular System*

Anaemia : Nasis Dam

Pale : Shahib

Oedema : Wethma

Blood Pressure Related Diseases

Hypertension : Irtifa Daght Addam.

Hypotension

Generalized : Umuman

Weakness Umumi : Dhuf, V. Yudhaif

Vertigo : Dukha

Vertige : Rasi ydoor

Gidiness : Dokha

Giddy : Dayikh

Headache ; Thuja : Waja Raas, Sudaa

Palpitations : Khafaqan

Postural Hypotension : Waqte Tabdil Taghyir, Badaala Youghayer : Hea : Mushkila

Heart Failure : Hubut Al Galb

Angina Pectoris : Addabha Assadria

Peripheral Vascular Diseases
: Varicose Veins;

Leg Varices : Addawali

Arteriosclerosis : Tasallub Assharayeen

Embolism : Aljalta Addamawiya

Thromboangitis : Buerger's Disease
Obliterans

Claudication Distance ; : Thuja, Huja Alam
Waja :Bedein : Kam **Geddas** :Masafa (Distance)

Reynold's Disease : Touch, Touching (Pathetic);
Jas, Yajlis, Mess, Yamiss,
Lemes Yilmas ; Mueththir

VII. *Dentistry*

Chew : Alas, Yalas, V. Madagh

Saliva : Riq, Luab

Wisdom Tooth : Sin El Ahle

Molar : Iddirse, Dhirs, Pl. Dhurus

Abscess : Indikhorag

Colloquial : Habba

Toothache : Wajsin (N)/Thuja, Huja,Alam Waja :
Asnan, Pl. Isnan

VIII. _Gastrointestinal System_

Digest, Digestion : Mulakh Khas, Zibda, Hadhham, Hadhmtaam

Dyspepsia : Usr Hadm

Hiccough : Bufag, Bilfag

Belching : Tagriaa

Distension : Intifah

Ulcer : Dumla, Karaha

Hyperacidity : Zaid Hamuda

Heart Burn : Gaddad

Haematemesis : Yiruddam

Melena : Batni Tigri Biddem

Constipation : Imesac, Qabudhiya

Diaorrhoea : Isaehaal, Ishal

Dysentery : Ishaldem, Dizanteri

Dehydration : Nagis Mayya

Haematemesis : Yirudam

Gall Bladder, Bile : Meeraash, Marrara, El Murrarrah

Stone : Ershad, Haswa, N.(Mineral) Hajar, Pl. Hijar, Debb Min Halquh

Vomitting : Ekdif, Radda, Kaei, Yazuu, Yazu, Yastafrigh, Taqqaya,Istafaragh

Nausea : Gafayan, Laben Nefs

Nauseate : Yulalib, Laben Nefs

Pain : Thuja, Huja, Alam, Waja

Colic: Maksha; Abdominal Colic: Batni Tilwi

Where : Wain, Wen, En, Menain

Severity Severe : Shadid; Less: Aaqal;
Continuous: Daiman, Kull Waqt; **Often**: Kathir Marrat,
Wajid; **Sometimes**: Badh Waqt, Waqti, Fourie.

Previous History : Gabl, Sabiq, Qabal (Previous)

Severe, How Many Times : Shadeed : Kam, Geddas

Radiation To Rt.Shoulder Back : Tahwil, Tabdil
:Ameenak Katif : Dahree, Dhahr

Relation To Fatty

Meals : Badein; Sameen Taam, Ekl, Manjariya

Fissure; Tear : N. Shaqq

Fistula : Nasur, Rishah

Sentinel Pile (Tag) : No Bachi, Pl. No Bachiya

Pain, Bleeding : During, : Thuja, Nezf ; Waqte, Fithna

With After Stool Badein ; Gabl ; Bourass, Gaeit

Flatus : Gazat

Haemorrhoids : Bawaseer, Pl. Basur, Khafir

Ascitis : Sagia

Cirrhosis : Teleyifal Kabid

IX. *Genitourinary System*

Sex : Jins

Eunuch : Khasi Pl. Khisyan, Mukshi, Makhasi

Puberty : Sinn El Bulugh

Precocious Puberty : Pulug Mubakkir

Delayed Puberty : Bulug Mutaakhir

Reproduction : Tanasul

Fertility : Khusb

Fertile : Mukhsib

Sterile (Of Woman) : Aqir

Impotence : All Ajiz, Daaf Jins

Impotent : Ajiz

Intercourse : Mukhalata, Muashra

Weak Erection : Nafsi Markhiyya

Nocturnal Emission : Gathaf Laili

Masturbation : Istimna

Syphlis : Frengi, Zuhriya, Zuhri

Venerial Diseases : Marad Tanasul

Conceive : Habalat, Tahbal

Pregnancy : Haml

Pregnant : Hamil

Labour : Wadhaa

Child Birth : Wilada

Normal Delivery : Wilada

Operation : Caesarian

Placenta : Khilas

Pueperium : Nifas

Abortion : Ijhaz, Ramu

Children : Alawlaad, Bambino

Number : Kam, Geddas

Elder : Kabir

Youngest : Saghir

Age : Umr (Colloquial)

Menstruation : Masaha, Dhaura, Haydhn,

Menarchae : Awal Marra ; (Menstruation) Aadah ; Umr

Menopause : Akhiran; Wagf Alhaydha

Menstrual Cycle :
Periodical Duration : Min Waqt, La Waqti ; **Flow** ;
Mudda, **Duration** :**Normal**, Akhtar **(Increase), (Less)**
Aqal
Dymenorrhoea

:Thuja**(Pain);**Waqte;Ithna;**(Mensruation)**

Irregularity : Adm Tertib **Irregular** : Min Dun Tertib,
Teshewsh Alaada
Vaginal Discharge : Madda Min Almahbil

X. *Urinary System*

Urine : Bool

Urinate : Bal, Yabul

Urgency : Dharura

Urge : Lahh, Ala, Yaluhh

Urodyanamics; Flow, : Jara, Yijri (Flow)

Stream Pressure : Pressing ; Dharuri, Lahh, Yaluhh
Flow, Stream Bad;

Flow, Stream : **(Improvement/Gone)** Mufid,Islah,
Taqaddum/Kharban

Nocturnal Frequency : Tabawul Laili, Kathir
Marrat Bool Wahed Lail

Dysuria : Harakan Al Bawl

Haematuria : Bouli Ahmar, Yibul Dam

Burning Micturition : Bouli Yuhrig, Harara Bool

Enuresis : Tabawul Lairadi

Circumcision : Tuhur, Tahhar, Khitan

XI. *Hernia*

Hernia : Fateigh, Fataq, Fatig, Ayyan

Reduciblity : **During, After, Strain, Size Increase**;

Waqte, Fiithna **(After)** Badein : Masha **(Movement),**

Shughl **(Work),** Riyadha **(Exercise)** : Kabir, Halba **(**
Colloquial**)**

During Lying Down : Reduce Waqte Fithna : Uru
Gudh, Nam Yanam :Daakhil Batn

Obstruction : Mani ; La Masha Daakhil Batn :

Problem : Before : Treatment

XII. *Paediatrics*

Foetus : Jenin

Infant : Radii

Infancy : Sughr

Baby : Radd

Adolescent : Baligh

Child : Walad, Pl. Awlad

Cry : Weep ; Beka : Siyah, Surakh

Weeping : Buka, Bucha

Feed : Tam, Tatam, Yutaim,Yatatam

Suckle : Radhdha, Yuradhdhi

Wean : Fatam, Yaftam

Weaning : Mafatoom

Malnutrition : Nagis Taghdia

Marasmic : Masrub

XIII. *Orthopaedics*

Sprain : Fesekh, Yifasakh

Fracture : Kasoora

Dislocation : Khalaa Fakke

Swelling : Waram, Wurum

Restriction : Movement; Tahdid : Haraka, Pl. Harakat

Amputate : Gass, Yaguss

Rickets : Kusah

Physiotherapy : Riyadha

Move : Harrak, Yuharrik

XIV. *Dermatology, Skin*

Mushkila Jild, Jilud

Sense of Touch : Lems

Birth Mark : Wahma

Naevus, Mole : Wahamah

Acne : Daamil

Ulticaria : Hassasiye

Sun Burn : El Tee Habel Gild

Skin Rash : Tafh Jildi

Prickly Heat : Hab Arag

Itching, Pruritus : N. Hakka, Hakkan, V.Hakk.Yahukk

Scabies : Al Jarab

Eczema : Hazaza

Wart : Talul

Psoriasis : Assadfiye

Leucoderma : Bahag

Vitiligo : Al Bahag

Leprosy : Bars, Leprus, Leper, Abras, Fem, Barsa, Pl. Burs, Bursin

Oriental Sore : Wagra

Lympthadenopathy : Tadakhum Gudad Allemf

Plague : Taun, Waba (Affliction), Dharba, Pl. Dharabat

Burn : Ahraq, Yuhriq, Ihtaraq, Yahtariq

Blister : Fasfoosa

Scab : Gishr

Scar : Kedema

Wrinkle : Tarqa

Polyhydrosis : Kathir Al Arag

CHAPTER—6
Medical History

History suggestive of Diabetes, Hypertension, Jaundice, Tuberculosis have been discussed with Endocrines (Thyroid), Cardiovsascular System (CVS), Gastrointestinal System (GIT), Respiratory System, Respectively

(A) History Suggestive of Allergy

Allergy : Mushkila Asabiya, Hassasiya

Cause Reason : Sebeb, Pl. Asbab

Known : Maruf, Yaref

Previous Treatment : Gabl, Qabal, Sabiq Elaaz

Details.

Duration.

Seasonal, Variation : (Season, Climate) Hawa,

Manakh, Fasl, (Variation)Ikhtilaf, Taghayyur

When : Amta

(B) History Suggestive Of Previous Surgery

(Previous) Gabl, Qabal, Sabiq ; **(Surgery)** Amaliyyah,

Jiraha, Dar Amaliyaah

Indication Surgery ;Why : Lesh, Laysh, Leemaatha;**(Surgery)**
Problem, Name For : **(Problem, Name)** Ismak
Purpose Duration. Mushkila, **(For)** Lee, **(Purpose)** Qasd, Ghaya, **(Surgery)**

Previous Treatment Papers : Gabl, Qabal, Sabiq (Previous)Warga Elaaz

Where : Wain, Wen, En, Menain

History Suggestive Of Other Problems : **(Is)** Fee ; **(Beside/other)**Tani, Gaadi, Akher, Akhar, F. Ukhra, Pl. Ukhar, Akhirin, Ghair ; **(Problem)** Mushkila

(C) *Family History*

Marriage : Zawaaj

Single : Ferd, Wahid

Unmarried : Azib

Married : Mutazzawaj, Mutehhel

Children : Bambino, Al Awlaad

Boy : Walad, Al Walad

Girl : Beinati

How Many : Kam, Geddas

Relation : Nisba

Relative : Nisbi

Father : Al Abb Colloquial : Baba

Mother : Al Umm Colloquial : Mama

(D) *Social History*

Smoker : Yudakkin, Dakhaan

Cigarettes : Jigara, Pl. Jigayir, Sebaas, Colloquial : Sipse

Cigar : Charut, Tuscani, Colloquial:Seghaayer

Tobacco : Titen, Dakhaan

Alcohol : Kuhool, Spirito, Wiski,Mashroobat

Other Intoxication : Akher, Akhar, F. Ukhar, Pl.

Ukhra, Akhirin Ghair; Sikr **(Intoxication)**

Duration Quantity : Miqdar, Kemmiya

(E) *Occupational History*

Profession : Mihnah

Occupation : Watheefa

Job : Amal, Shooghel

Military : Askari, N. El Askariya

CHAPTER—7
Clinical Examination

Examination : Imtihan; Fahs

Examine : Imtahan, Yamatahin, Fahas,Yifhas

Sign : Waqqa, Yuwaqqi, Alama, Plalamat

Request/Asking for: : Mumkin **(Possible)** ;
Shoof **Examination (Examine)**

Pulse (At Wrist) : Nabdh

**Blood Pressure; For Tying Blood Pressure
Instrument
Cuff, Removing Cloth Fold/Up; This** : **(Fold)** Tawa,
Yatwi/Foq; Hathe **(This)**

Temperature; Body : Derjetel Harara

Temperature Thermometre, : Thirmomethre Taht/Hadr/
Under the, Tongue Joa **(Under),** Lissan **(Tongue)**

Please : Fadlak (M), Fadlik (F). Colloquial : Fatdh, fatth (S)
;
Fadal, Fadhal (Pl.)

For Asking To Lie Down (Rest Horizontally) : Uru
Guuddh (Nam,Yanam, Nom)

Long : Taweel

Raise Lift Legs/ Shoulders/Head : Rafa, Yarfav V., Irfaa

Bend Flex; Knees :Limb (Extremity) : **(Bend)** Itney;
(Knees) Rukub, Rukabh ; Atraf :**(Foreleg) (Hind Leg)**
Dual

Deep: Breadth : **(Breath)** Teneffus, Nefs,
Nefes : Amiq **(Deep)**
Hold : Yemsik
Cough : Kahha, Gahha, Gahh, Yaguhh

Again : Min Jadeed, Colloquial :Marratania

Repeat : Kerrer, Youkarir (V.)

Open Mouth : **(Open)** Fetha, Iftah Fam **(Mouth)**

Close Mouth : Dhayyiq

Please, Show : Mumkin Shoof

Protrude Tongue : **(Protrude)** Tala; Yitla Lissan

(Tongue)

Please Show Teeth : Mumkin Shoof: Warini ;
Isnan, Acnanik

Say Aaa : Kalaam Aaa

Open Eyes : Iftah Ain (S) : Ayoun (Pl.)
Close Eyes : Dhayyiq, Bhamed : **Eyes**

Follow, This : **(Follow)** Ishbah, Teba Yitba: Hathe **(This)**

Look Up; Roof : **(Look up)** Shoof Foq ; Saqaf **(Roof)**

Look Down; Floor : **(Look Down)** Shoof Lowta;
Rakhees ; Tabeq **(Floor)**

Press; This : **(Press)** Shid, Asar, Yasar; Hathe **(This)**

Pull; This : **(Pull)** Iibid, Jarr, Jarara ;Hathe **(This)**

Push; This : **(Push)** Def, Defa ; Hathe **(This)**

This : Hathe (S.) (F.), Hatha (Pl.) (M.)

Internal; Examination : **(Internal)** Dakhili ; Imtihan/
Fahs **(Examination)**
Per Rectal : Bisharaj
Per Vaginal : Bilfam
Stand : Qif Yaqif (V.)
Stand Up : Qam, Yaqum

Thank You : Shukran

Thanks : Teshekkur, Shukr

Do Not Mention It : Afwan

Never Mind : Mahlesh

Do Not Bother : Mush Muhimmah

Please ; Go : **(Please)** ; Imshi Masha **(Go)**

CHAPTER—8
Investigations

Investigation, Analysis : Teftish, Tahqiq/Tahleel

Test : Imtihan, Tajriba

(I) Laboratory Investigations

Laboratory : Mamal : Ahwa, Yahwi **(Have Inside)
Container ;** Contain.

Tube : Lula (Of Metal, Andc.) / Teube

Blood Tests : Damm, Dem, Pl. Dima **(Blood)**

Variety; Group : Jamaa, Taskeela

Blood Test (N.) : Fahas Damm

Urine Tests:

Urine : Bool

Mid Stream Sample : 1. Urinate : Bal, Yabul
2. Mid : Nuss, Nusf/**Middle :**Wast, Mutawassit/
   Between : Ben, Maben;
3. Flow/Stream : Yizri/Zara
4. Container

Stool Tests; Stool : Buraas, Gaeit

Sputum Tests ; : Tefel, Yitfal, Nakhama (Sputum)

Semen Tests ; Mani **(Semen)**

Sperm : Hayawan, Manawi

Body Fluid Tests;

Biochemistry, Microscopy,

Pus Tests; Pus : Mudd, Jaraha

Germ : Jarthuma, Pl. Jarathim

Microbe : Mikrob

Sediment : Dihla

Culture, Senstivity Tests :

Culture : Thaqafa

Senstivity : Hassas

React : Radd, Yarudd

Appropriate : Adj. Muwafiq, Layiq, Munasib

Histopathology (Biopsy) : (After) Baad, Badein
(Surgery) Jiraha, Amaliyyah;**(Microscope)** Mukebbir,
Mijhar ; **(Test)**
Endoscopy : Mandaar

Sample, Specimen : Namuna, Pl. Namayin

II. *Radiodiagnosis*

Radiology X Ray : Suura, Eshia, Runtjeniya

Contrast Radiology : **(Colour)** Lon, Rang; **(X-Ray)**
Suura, Eshia

IVP : Intra Venous Pyelography : Suura Mulona

Retrograde : Ila Wara

Barium Study : Suura Gyps

Ultrasound : Zehaas

CT Scan : Computter ; X-Ray

III. *Non Invasive Procedures*

Doppler's

ECG ; Heart : Galb, Qalb, Tests

EEG ; Brain : Mukh, Dimagh, Tests

IV. *Invasive Procedures*

Endoscopy : Mandaar

1. GIT; Upper : Foqani, Foq. **Lower** : Nasi, Lowta.

2. Urology : Upper, Lower: Bawliyya, Masalak **(Urology)**

Result : Nateeza, Pl. Natayiz

Report : Taqrir, Raport

Normal : Adi, Tabee

CHAPTER—9
Diagnosis : Disease

Diagnosis : Tashkis

Disease : Waj, Awja Pl., Mardh, Pl.Amradh

Consultation : Mashwara

Advice, Opinion,

Suggestion : Nasiha, Pl. Nasayih, Rai, Pl. Ara, Fikr, Pl. Afkar, Eqtirrah

Various Diseases are Categorized as Congenital, Hereditary Traumatic Inflammatory, Infectious. (Specific)/(Non-specific), Neoplastic

Infectious : Contagious, Diseases ;
Sari, Mudi : Sari, **Diseases**

Arabic Expressions,
Inflammation : Iltihab, Inflammatory : Multehib, Prefixed or Suffixed to the Name of Body Organ, System Effected, Practically Serves the Purpose of Expression for Disease, Diagnosis of Inflammatory Category.

Other Common Diseases of Defferent Categories, Have Been Discussed With Clinical History, Symotomatology, of Various Body Systems, Respectively.

CHAPTER—10
Treatment
I. Medical Treatment

Medicine : Dawa, Pl. Edwiya
Dispensary : Mustawsaf
Pharmacy : Sedaliya
Pharmacist : Ejzachi, Pl. Ejzachiya

Quantity : Miqdar

Amount : Miblagh, Pl. Mabaligh,

TSF (Tea Spoonful)
Tea : Sagir
Table : Kabir
Spoon : Khashuga, Kashik

Tablet : Haboob, Qarsa, Pl. Quras

Capsule : Kabsula

S/L; Sub Lingual : Taht, Hadr, Joa : Lissan

Injections; Syringe : Sharqa, Haqna, Ibra, Shringa, Yibra

Needle : Ibra

Injection : Libra, Hugan

S/C, Subcutaneous ; : Taht Elzild
Hypodermic

I/M ; Intramuscular : Dakhil Adal, Feel Adal

I/V; Intravenous : Dakhil Irk

I/Arterial; Intrarterial : Dakhil Shoryaen

I/Vascular; Intravascular : Dakhil Damar, Fe El Reg

I/Cardiac Intracardiac : Dakhil Galb/Qalb

Vaccine : Laqah

Vaccination : Talqih

Immunity : Muaf **(From Sickness)** Manaa

A.S.T ; After

Senstivity Test : Badein Imtihan, Fahas, Tajriba

React : Radd, Yarudd

Senstivity : Hassas

Syrup : Dibes

Tonic : Muqawwi

TSF : **Table/Tea, Spoon, Full**

Drops : Katra

Oral : Sharab

Nasal : Li Lanf, Khashim/Khashm

Ointment : Marham, Dihn, Dehaan, Bumaata

Powder : Gubra, Budra

Lotion : Ghasil, Masah

Cream : Dahan

Massage : Ferk

Mouth Gargle : Gargara, Lilfam, **(Medicine)** Dawa

Rinse : Feyya, Yufeyyi, **(Medicine)** Dawa

Vapour : Bukhar

Spray : Bakh, Rash

Suppository : Zer Boot : Dakhil Sharaj Dawa,

Enema : Hukna Sharjiya, Traumba

Sitz's Bath :
Luke Warm : Fatir
Water : Mai, Emmaya, Maea
Medicine : Dawa, **Mixed (Compounded)** Makhlut,
Mamzuj/ **After Mixing** : Badein Youkhalet(V.)
Container : **Tub** : Hodh/Hamam
Sit : Gaams/Qaad, Yaqad/Jeles, Yizlas
Ten/Fifteen ; Minutes : A s h r a a / K h a m s t a a s h
Khamsataash ; Daqeeqa/Digheegha (Minutes)

Once A Day : Wahed Marra Faqat Wahed
Youm/Youm, Wahed Marra/Merra Fi El Youm
Twice A Day : Youm Zouz : Etnain Marra/ Marra Zouz :
Etnain Youm/Merratyen Fi El Youm
Thrice A Day : Telaeta Marra Kull Youm/
Youm Telaeta Marra/Thlath Mrat Fi El Youm
Four Times A Day : Arba Marra Kull Youm/
Youm Arba Marra/Arba Merra Fi El Youm

Every Hour : Kull Saa

Every Week ;Once A Week : Wahed Marra/Marra
Wahed : Esboo/Marra Fi El Asboaa/
Marra Wahed; Esboo Wahed

Hour of Sleep : Waqte Noum, Indannawn

Stat ; Immediately : Bisaaa, Hessa, Halan,

Without Anything Intervening : Min Dun Wasita

Stat And Once, Only : Halan Wa/Miya Marra

Wahed, **(Only)** Faqat, Baas

Stat And SOS : Halan Wa/Miya Waqte Lazem/Indalluzum
SOS : Waqte Lazem/Indalluzum

Alternate Day : Youm Baad Youm
Before ; Meals : Gabl, Sabiq, Qabl
Food : Taam, Ekl
Breakfast : Futur
Supper : Ashaa
Dinner : Gazaa
After Meals : Baad Badein : **Meals : Food**
With : Meals ; Maa, Wiya : Meals : Food
Duration ; Treatment : Kam Youm, Kam Waqt,
Geedas Waqt ; **(Treatment)**Elaaz
O.D : Once A Day : (☐)
B.D : Twice A Day : (☐) (☐)
T.D.S : Thrice A Day : (☐) (☐) (☐)
Q.I.D : Four Times A Day : (☐) (☐) (☐) (☐)
H.S : Hour Of Sleep
A. D : Alternate Day
P.C : After Meals
Stat : Immediately
SOS : If Need
Due Precaution has to be taken, for Drug Schedule,
Explanation and or Administration to the Patient,
Assisted by Pharmacist and Nursing Staff.

(II) Surgical : Jarahi

Surgery : Jiraha, Amaliyyah

Surgeon : Jarrah

Decide : Azam, Yazam

Surgery : Necessary : Jiraha, Amaliyyah : Lazim, Lazm, Dharuri, Thuroory

Timely : Fi Waqtuh

Pre Operative Patient : **Consent** : Ridha

Grave (Of Illness) : Increase : Risk : Consent ; Mukhtir : Izdiyad, Ziyada, Halba : Mukhatara : Ridha

Surgery Preparation : Youjahiz (V.) Sabab Amaliyyah

Part Preparation, Shave, Shaving : Remove Hair : Zayan : Shal, Yashil, Vaqal,Yanqal Shar

Nil Per Oral (N. P. O.), : La Shafahi, Nusf El Lel,Nuss El **Midnight** Lel, Nesf Al Lail

After : Baad, Badein

Anaesthetist Consultation : Doctorr Takhdir, Mashwara

Post Operative Patient Observation

Watch Vitals : Nadhr, Temyiz, Mutebih, Ainala : Muhim.

Insert : Dakhkhal, Yudakhkhil

Flatus : Gazat

Take Turn : Tabdil, Taghyir, Baadaala, Youghayer : Hea

Postural Positional Changes : Mawqa, Pl. Mawaqi, Makan,
Pl. Amakin

Condition : Hal, Pl. Ahwal

Good : Kuways, Tayyib, Pl.Tayyibin, Zen, Pl. Zenin, N. Surur

Satisfactory : Hasab Al Murad, Ala Kef

Normal : Adi

Status Quo : Al Hala Kema Hiya

Discharge Advice : Tejenneban, Yetejenneb

Avoid ; Forbidden : Mamnu, Yasaq

Dressing, Bandage : Laffafa, Rabat, Shedda, Riyar, Fasha, Robat Shaesh,

Removal Withdraw : Naqal, Yanqal, Jarr, Yajurr, Barra.

Alternate Day : Youm Baad Youm.

Every Day : Kull Youm.

Follow Up Come Back , : Raja, Yarja, Ruju ; Taal,

Return : Hospital ; Maasha **(Come Back)** ; Mustashfa

(Hospital); Baad, Badein **(After)** ; Kam/ Geddas **(How many)** ; Youm **(Duration)**

CHAPTER—11
Paramedical Staff

Nurse : N. Mudaria, Pl. Mudariyat, V. Dara, Yudari

Nurse Male : Mamarridh

Nurse Female : Mamarridha

Matron : Raisat Mumarridhat

Technician : Fanni

Radiology Technician : Fanni Ashiaa

Laboratory Technician : Fanni Maamal

Anaesthesia

Technician : Fanni Takhdir

Physiotherapist Technician : Fanni Ilaj Tabii

Assistant Pharmacist : Masaid Saydali

Midwife : Obstetrics Gynaecology, Nurse : Kabilah :
Mamarridh (M.) Mamarridha (F.) Nissa Wilada

Operation Theatre : **Technician**; Fanni,
Mamarridh (M.), Mamarridha (F.) : Jarrah, Jiraha,
Amaliyyah, Dar Amaliyaah

Nursing Staff

Torch : Battariyya

Help : Musada, Yousaad

Nurse : V. Dara, Yudari, N.Mudaria, Pl. Mudariyat

Male Nurse : Mamarridh

Female Nurse : Mamarridha

Matron : Rai Sat Mumarridhat

Preparation; Bed : **(Preparation)** Istidad,Yuhadhdhir, Youjahiz (V.) ;Sareer, Firash, Fraash **(Bed)**

Pillow : Makhadda, Pl. Makhadit

Pillow Case : Wajh Makhadda

Blanket : Planket, Pl. Planketat, Hram, Pl. Hramat

Sheet : Charchaf, Pl. Charachif

Observation, Watch Vitals : As : Adv. : Nadhr, Temyiz, Mutebih Ainala Muhimm : Mithl : Nasiha, Pl. Nasayih

Medicine, Refuse : Yarfuth (V.)

Positional Postural Changes, Take Turn : Baadaala, Tabdil, Taghyir, Youghayer, Hea, Mawqa, Pl. Mawaqi, Makan, Pl. Amakin

Transfer, Shift Patient : **(Transfer, Shift)** N. Tahwil, Hawwal, Yuhawwil, Naqal, Yanqal ; **(Patient)** Mareeth, Mareedh, Pl. Mardha

71

Operation Theatre Staff

Surgery : Jiraha, Amaliyyah

Surgeon : Jarraha

Operation Theatre : Dar Amalliyah **(OT)**
Fanni;**Technician (Nurse, M. F.)**

Sterlization : Taqim

Sterlize : Tahhar, Yutahhir, Naqqa,Yunaqqi, Aqqam

Sterile (Disinfected) : Muaqqam

Disinfectant : Muaqqim

Fumigation : Tabkhir

Fumigate : Yubakhir, Bakhkhar

Infection : Isaba, Tesemmum

Equipment : Adawat, Muhimmat,Muaddaat

Instrument : Ala, Pl. Alat, **(Means)** Wasita, Pl. Wasayit

The need arising during various occasions, to complete clinical examination, investigative procedures, during treatment : Medical, Surgical, Physiotherapy, can be satisfied by Arabic Translation of the Expressions;

Do : Sawwa, Yusawwi.

Like This : Mutashaabih Hatha (M.) (Pl.), Hathi(F.) (S.), Hichi Hakadha;

Similar, Same : As That : Mithl, Yishbah, Hadhak, Dhak

72.

CHAPTER—12
Medical Specialists

General Practitioner : Tabib Aam

Surgeon : Jarrah, Tabib Jiraha

Physician : Tabib, Pl. Atibba

Internist : Tabib Batini

Paediatrician : Tabib Atfal

Gynaecologist : Tabib Nissa

Obstetrician : Tabib Wilada

Urologist : Tabib Bawliyya, Masalak

E.N.T. Specialist : Tabib Anf Wa Udun Wa Hunjurah

Opthalmologist : Tabib Uyun

Dermatologist : Tabib Jildiyya

Dentist : Tabib Asnan

Orthopaedist : Tabib Izam

Physiotherapist : Tabib Ilaj Tabii

Radiologist : Tabib Ashiaa

Anaesthetist : Tabib Takhdir

Neurologist : Tabib Aasaab

Psychologist : Tabib Amrad Nafsiya

Pharmacist : Tabib Saydali

Veterinarian : Tabib Baytari

Veterinary Surgeon : Betar

Medical Jurist : Tabib Sharii

Medical- : Tubbi ; Fiqh

Juris prudence

Arabic expression of concerned Anatomical Organ,

System, When Prefixed or Suffxed to, Doctor

Colloquial : **Doctorr, Practically Serves the Purpose,**

For Arabic Expression of, Dealing Medical Specialist.

PART-(2)
CONTENTS

'Supplement : Common Use Arabic'

                                                    Page

I. Useful Arabic Expressions
   (A) Introductory 77
   (B) Understanding Language 80
   (C) Official 82
   (D) Usful Phrases
       Useful Vocabulary 85

II.Useful Grammar 102

III. Time, Week Days, Months, Seasons 113
     Cardinal Points, Colours,
     Human Relations Etc

CHAPTER—I
Useful Arabic Expressions

(A) Introductory

Peace be Upon You : Assalam alay-kum

In Reply : Wa alay-kum assalam

Good morning : Sabah-al-khair, Sabbhakum
Allah Bil Khair

Good evening : M'sà-al'khair

Good night : Amsà-ala-khair (m)
Amsi-ala-khair (f)
Good night everyone : Amsoo-ala-khair (pl)

Hello ! : Ahlan-wa-sah-Ian

How are you? : Kaif-halak (m) Kaif-halik (f)

I am well : Taib (m) Taiba (f), Kuweis (m) Kuweisah (f)

Thank-you : Shukran

And You How are You?: Wa anta keif-haalak (m)
Wa anti keif-haalik (f)

Not so bad : Mush Battaal

How do you do? : Fursa-saeeda (or) Ahlan-wa-sah-an

You are welcome : Ahlan-wa-sah-an

What is the matter? : La-baas (or) Shinu-fee

Yes : Na-am

This is a... : Hatha (m) Hathi-hi (f)

Congratulations : Mab-rook (m & f)

Cheers! : Fee sahattak? (m)

Happy birthday : Eed-meelaad saeed

Happy feast : Eed-saeed

Happy anniversary : Kul-sana wa-anta tà yeb(m)

The same to you : Shukran

Allow me to introduce..: Asmah-li oorefak
... you to Mr. : Bissayed...

Pleased to see you : Forsa-saeeda

Will you please? : Min-fadlak (m) Min-fadlik (f)

Excuse me : An-ith-nak (m), An-ith-nik (f)

Very Sorry : **(Sorry)** Aasif (m), Aasifa (f), **(very)** Jiddan

Regret, Regret very : Mu-Ta-Assif (m),

Much Mu-ta-assifa (f)

Not at all, Do not Mention it, I beg your pardon : Af-

wan

Really : Haqeqatan

Good : Kuwais (m) Kuwaisa (f)

Bad : Mush kuwais (m) Mush kuwaisa (f)

Good gracious (oh dear) : Ya salaam!

Cheer up! : Af-rah

Never mind : Ma-aleish, Ma-eehemsh

Please : Min-fadlak (m) Min-fadlik (f)

77

What is the matter? : La-baas (or) Shinu-fee?

Nothing. : La-shai (or) Ma-feeshai

I think so : Youmken (or) Mumkin

I do not think so : Mush mumken

You are right : Andak hagh

Very well : Ta'yeb (or) Kuwais

Give my regards to... : Balligh Salaami ila ...

By chance : Be-assood-fa

Don't worry : La tash-ghool baalak (m)

By all means : Ya-salaam tafaddal

Certainly : Tab-an

I am very sorry : Muta-assef jiddan

(B) Understanding Language

Do you understand me? : Fe-hem-ti-nee (m)
Fe-hem-tee-nee (f) Fe-hem-too-nee (pl)

I do not understand you : Ma-naf-hamsh eish taghool

What do you want? : Maatha tureed? (m)

Do you speak English? : ta-ref inghileesi?

I do not speak Arabic : Man-takallmsh Arabi
But I am learning it : Walakan ghaa-ad-nataallum,
(learn) taallam, yata' allam; arabi

I hope to learn it quickly: Insha allah nata allam-ha

feesa

Speak slowly : So that I can understand
you : Ta-kalem bish-waish Baish naghdar nafhmak

We need an Interpreter?: Eh-nah ow-zeen mu-tar-Gim,
(interpreter);tarjaman, tarjamaniya (fl)

You have to answer in Arabic: Anta yajib an tarudd bi
al-arabi anta **(you)** jawab,yujawib **(answer)** al-arabic,
arabic faqt **(in arabic only)**

Dictionary : Qamu, Qawamis (pl.)
(Words available); Kalimat

Vocabulary : Muf-Raadaat

How do you say this in Arabic? : Kaif T-ghool haatha Bil Arabee?

Do you understand this? : Hal anta fahami hatha?

Is this understood by you : Hal hatha mafhoom?

I do not konw : La-aref, ma-na-refish, ehnahmish ahrfeen   **(Imagine)**

I believe so : Ata-qid hakada

I Imagined so : Tassawwara hakatha
Tasawwar,
Yatasswar, takhayyal,yatakhayyal

Will you Help me? : Saa-idni min-fathlak (m)
Saa-idni min-fathlik (f)

Allow me to help you : Asmah-li en-saadak (m)

Can I help you? : Hal-mumken ensaadak?(m)

It is impossible : La-youmken

It is not possible : Mush mumken

Please yourself : Anta wa shaanak (m)

As you like : Keif ma tahib (or) T-reed

Allow me : Asmah-li (m)

(C) Official

What is your name? : Shinu asmak (m),Ismaak (m.s),
Shinu asmik (f),Ismik (f.s)

My name is .... : Ana/sme......, / sme.......

And what is yours? : Wa eish ismak (m),Ismik (f)

Write your name : Iktib asmak (m) Iktibi asmik (f)

How old are you? : Kam umrak? (m)

What is your address? : Shenu an-waanak?

That's it : Kuwais (or) Baahee

It is too much : Waajid (or) Katheer

Place of birth : Makaan al-welaadah

Nationality : al-jensiya

Marital status : Al-haala al-ij-teemaaiya

Single or married : Aazeb aw mutazawej

Salary required : Aazeb aw mutazawej

Are you now employed: Hal-tash-taghel tawa?

What is your education? : Shenu taleemak?

Is it primary? : Hal huwa ib-teedaee?

Preparatory : Ee-daadi

Secondary : Tà-nawi

Have you any degrees?: Hal andak shahadaat ul-ya?

Where were you employed? : Wain kunt tash-taghel?

What is the reason for leaving? :
Shenu sabab tar'k al-amall?

For salary reasons : Al-asbaab heya arrateb

I would like to see Mr. : Mumken enshoof essayed..

He is not in at the moment :
Huwa mush maw-jood, tawa

He will be here at ... : Yar-jaah essa-a...

Come and visit me at home : Ta-aal (or) Tafathal zoor-ni
fee al-beit

When? : Amta?

Any time you like : Fee ay waqt t-heeb (or)Tureed

Then I'll come to see you in the afternoon :
Emmala enjee enshoofak ba-ad ath-hur

Is that alright? : Hal anta mu-wafaq?

Of course : Tab-ann (or) Aywa

Splendid (great) : Atheem

How do you go there? : Ah-rroh he-nak iz-zi?

Do you know the way? : Ta-ref attareegh? (m)

Show me the street : Warreeni asharea (m)

Do you live here? : Hal-teskun hana? (m)

This is my house/office : Hatha beity (or) Man-zali

I live here : Ana nas-kun hana

Have you got a car? : Hal andak sayyara?

No, sorry : La aasef

But that isn't a problem : Walakin hathi mush mush-kila

I'll get my friend's car : Sa-na-khuth sayyarat Sadeeqi

Can you come back tomorrow?: Taghdar (or) mumken tar-jaah buchra?

Agreed, I'll see you next Friday : Attafaq-na sa-antatharak
youm ajjuma al-muq-bila

I hope : En-sha-allah

Don't forget the appointment : Ma-tan-saash al-maw-ed

I hope not : En-sha allah là

Good bye : Maa-assalaama (or) Biassalaama

Appointment : Al-maw-ed

Visit : Yazoor (v), ziyara, Pl.ziyarat

Signature : Taw-qeea, Imdha, Alama,Pl. alamat

Director : Al-Moodeer

Cause : Sebeb, Pl. Asbab

Care : Iteni, Ihtemm, Yehtemm,

Caution, Take Care; Taqayyad

Vain, Useless : Abath, Abathan, Bila Fayida

(D) <u>Usful Phrases</u>

Come in : Ta-aal (or) Ud-Khal

Come quickly : Taal-bisur-aa (m)

I don't care a bit : La yahummuni abadan

Where are you going? : Wain maashi? (m)

Please come here : Min-fathlak ta-aal hana

Please go there : Min-fathlak emshi hanaak

Just a minute : Lah-tha minfath-lak

Please sit down : Tafadal ejles (m) Tafadli ejlesi (f)

May I see you? :
Mumkin enshoofak (m)Mumkin enshoofik (f)

Of course, please do : Tab-ann-tafathal

How are you feeling now? : Kaif sah-ttak tawa? (m)
Kaif sah-ttik tawa? (f)

Make tea : Deer shahee (m)

Make coffee : Deeri ghah-wa (f)

Switch off the light : Tafee a-nnoor (m)

Put on the light : Walla-ee a-nnoor (f) Walla a-nnoor (f)

Turn off the radio : Tafee a-rradiu (m)

What is this? : Shinu hatha? (m)

What is that? Ay Da? : Shinu hatha? (m)

How much is this? : Bikam hatha? (m)

What have you got? : Maatha andak? (m)

There is a great difference Between them:

Fee far-gh kabeer: Ma bayn-hum

For (because) : Ala shaan

Do you mind if I sit down?: Hai-tass-mahli naghud al kursi?

I listen to you : Ana an-sut ilaik (m)

I am hearing you : Ana as-maa-feek (m)

I am ready : Ana jaahiz

I have no time : Ma-andish waqt

Behind time : Muta-akher

A bit at a time : Qaleelan qaleelan

There is some tea : Fee esh-waya shaahi

In the kitchen : fee al-mat-bakh

But there isn't any milk : Wa-laakin ma-feesh ay
(or) wala haleeb

Desk : Taa-wla, pl. taw-laat

Black Board : Saboora pl. sabooraat

Repeat, it please : Bitool aymin fadlak (m)
bitool aymin fadlik (f)(repeat); kerrer, yukerrir,youkarir (v)

Grocer
(Baqqal, Pl. Baqaqil)

Beans : Fassooliya

Biscuits : Bash-koot

Broad beans : Fool

Butter : Zubda, Zibed

Cheese : Jub-na, ziben

Coffee : Ghah-wa

Flour : Daqeeq (or) Taheen

Egg(s) : Baitha(s), dahruja, pl. dahard

Grain : **(In bulk);** taam, habubat, **(single seed)** : habba, pl.hubub habba ya, pl. habbayat

Honey : Asall

Lentils : Adass, ades

Macaroni : Macaroona, maka rana

Marmalade : Ma'joon (or) Murabba, marabba purtgal

Milk : Haleeb

Oil : Zait, dihnzet **(olive oil),** dihnkharwa **(castor oil)**

Olive : Zaitoon

Peas : Bezilya, humus

Pepper : Filfill

Rice : Rezz, timmen, snileb

Salt : Melah, milh

Soap : Saboon

Sugar : Sukker (or) Succar

Tea : Shahee **(tea pot);** kuri, **(tea cup);** finjan, pl. fanajin

Tin of Tomatoes : Ulba-tamaatem

Vinegar : Khall

Baker
(Khabbaaz, Pl. Khabbazin)

Fresh Bread : Eish

Loaf of Bread : Regifeish

Butcher
(Jajjaar, Gassab, Pl. Gasasib)

Lamb : Kharoof

Meat : La-ham

Veal or Beef : Laham bagaar (or) Ea-jel

Mince meat (ground beef) : Laham maf-room

Chops or cutlets : Kharoof

Fillet steak : Shareehat Iaham baqar

Leg of lamb : Fakh-that-kharoof

Kidney : Kilwa(s) kilaawi (pl)

Chicken : Dajaaja(s) Dajaaj (pl)

Fish Monger
(Hawaat, Baayasamak)

Fish : Samak

A fish : Samaka, Semcha

Fresh : Taa-za, Tazi, Tari, Jadid

Not fresh : Mush-taa-za, atiq

Fisherman : Sayyadsemek, pl. sayadin

Green Grocer
(Khathaar, Baqqal, Pl. Baqaqil)

Almonds : Louz

Apricots : Mish-mish

Apples : Attufah, tuffaha

Bananas : Al-banaani (or) Mouz

Beans (green) : Fasoolya khath-ra

Cauliflower : K-ramb (or) Kar-nabeet

Carrots : Jazer, Juzr

Chestnuts : Ghastal (or) Gastal

Cucumber : Kheeyaar

Dates : Tamar or Balah, tamra

Dried onions : Basal yaabis

Egg Plant : Badenjaan

Figs : Al-teen, tina, pl. tin

Fruits(s) : Faakiha(s) Fawaakih(pl)

Garlic : Thoom (or) Toom

Grapes : Al-anab, **(Grape-vine)**; tislaga, asmaya

Green onions : Basal khathar

Lemons : Al-limoon

Lettuce : Khass (or) Salaata

Melon : Batteekh

Nuts : Louz

Okra : Baamya

Onions : Basal

Oranges : Al-burtu-ghaal, portugala, pl. portugal

Peaches : Al-khookh

Pears : Al-kometra

Peas : Bezilya

Pomegranates : Rommaana(s) Rommaan (pl)

Parsley : Maa-danoos

Potatoes : Bataats

Radish : Fajal

Strawberries : Faraw-lah

Tomatoes : Tamaatem

Turnips : Lift

Water melon : Batteekh, reggi

Hotel
(Loqanda, Otel)

I would like a single room :
Enreed hujra li shakhis wahed
Double room : Enreed hujra muz-dawij,
(double); qaten, mudhaaf
The hotel : Al-hootell (or) Al-funduq

The manager : Al-moodeer

Enquiries : Ista-Iamaat

The porter : Al-bawaab, hammal, pl.hamamil

The waiter : Asuf-raaji, **(at table)**;sufrachi

The lounge : Assaala

Laundery : Ghassala, maghsal, hudum elghasil

The dining room : Saalet al-akel, sufra khana

The bedroom : huj-rat annoum, manam, gubat nom

The key : Al-muftaah, miftahi pl.mifatih

The first floor : Attabic al-awel

The bathroom : Al-hammaam

Call me at ... : Naadeeni anda ...

7 o'clock : Assa-a sab-à

I would like to ... : Enreed (or) Nebbi ...

Change my room : En-ghayer huj-rati

I shall be back : Sanar-ja

Late : Muta-akher

Early: : Muba-kir

Room No. : Rakkem el-huj-ra

Have you any letters? : Hal-lee-risaayel?

Message : Risaala (or) Mukaalema

For me : Lee-ana

Room : Hujra, gurfa, pl. ghuraf

Luggage : Haqaayeb (or) Shanaati

Bring the bags : Jeeb al-haqaayeb

I shall leave the hotel : Nebbi net-rek al-funduq

At dawn : Anda al-fajer

In the morning : Fee assabaah

At noon : Fee nesf annahaar

My bill please : Hesaabi min-fad-lak

Host : Sahib El Mahall

Hostile : Mudhadd, Dhudd

Hurt : E-wajah, waj, awwar, yuawwir

Restaurant
(Loqanida)

The menu : Qaayemat al-akel (or)At-taam

May I have : Mumken-ta-teeni

Mineral water : Maya-ma-danya

I should like : Nebbi (or) Enreed

Are you serving : Hal al-ghadaa

Table for two please : Ta-wala lit-nain min naas min-fadlak

Special dish : Ta-aam khusoosi

Sandwich : Sandwish

Spoon : Kaashik

Fork : Shauka

Knife : Moos (or) Sekeen

Plate : Soonya(s) Suwaani (pl)

Glass : Kubbaya (or) Taasa

May I have : Ateeni min-fadlak

May we have : Ateena min-fadlak

Some Water : Shewaya Maya

Nothing more : La-shai aakhar

Hot water : Maya sakh-na

Cold water : Maya ber-dà

Open (command) : Af-tah

Close : Sakker (or) Agh-fell

Go : Emshi (m & f), Mesha

Call a taxi : Naadili taaxee

Where is the ... : Wain al ...

Telephone : Talafoon (or) Al-haatif

W.C. : Beit-arraha (or)Al-hammam

Lift : Mis-add, (elevator): Jarr athqal

Cafe : Maq-haa, ga-hwa

Have you newspapers?: Andakum jaraayed?

Dinner (Noon meal, Lunch) : Tataghadda(v) Ghadà (n)

Dinner? (Evening) : Tata-ashaa(v) Ashaa (n)

Breakfast : Tef-tar(v) Futoor(n), Rayuq

Travel
(Sefer, Siyaha, Youssaafir (v))

My name is... : Ismee...

I would like to book for.. : En-reed neh-jezz lee...

Ticket : Tath-kira, teskera, pl.tasakir

For tomorrow : Lee-bukraa

For next week : Lee-ass-boo almuq-bal

When does the plane depart?: Amta etsaafer attayera?
(Departure); rawah

When does the plane arrive? : Amta tu-sill attayera?
(arrival); wasal

Telll me the flight number : Ghool-lee raqam arrih-la

Is there a bus? : Andakum auto-bees?

The bus is fully booked : Al-auto-bees mah-jooz

My telephone number is... : Raqam talafooni ...

Best car : Ah-san sayyara

Transport : Yan-qul (v), Naqliya (n) Naqal, Yanqal

Out of Reach : Ma-yaanash

Petroleum : Gaz. nafadh, dihn

Airport

Aeroplane : Taayaara, pl. taayaarat

International : Du-waly

Airport : Mataar El-cahira, minajovi

Vaccination : Ta-eem, tal-qih

Certificate : Shahaada

Passport : Jawaaz-safr

Visa : Tà-heera

Entry : Du-khool, madkhal

Exit : Khu-rooj

The customs : Al-jamaaregh, resm, pl. rusnmat

Custom house : Gumruk

Suitcase or briefcase : Shanta (f)

Box : Sanduq, pl. sanadiq

handbag : Shantat-yad

This is my bag : Hadi-he shanti, **(bag)**; kis,pl. akyas

This not mine : Hathe-mush-lee

How many bags ... : Kam shanta ...

... do you have : ... Andak (m) (s)

One bag : Shanta waheda

Two bags : Shantatain

Three bags : Talaata shanaatee

Please open your bag : Min-fad-lak aftah ashanta
Have you anything to declare? : Hal-andak ay-shai?
(Declare); alan, yulin
I have nothing to declare : Ma-andish-shai

I have some gifts : Andi ba-ath hadaaya lee shakhseeyan, (gift); hadiya,pl. hadaya

It is already opened : Maf-tooh

I have : Andi

Cigarettes : Sebaasi (or) Seghaayer jigara, pl. jigayir

Cigars : Tus-caani, charut

Perfume : Ra-waayah, atr

I have no... : Ma-andish

... Spirits : Kuhool

Liqueurs : Mash-roobaat

Tobacco : Dakhaan

Jewellery : Jawaaher, (ornament); zina

That is all I have : Hada ma andi

Here is my passport : Tafadal jawaaz safari, **(passport);** teskera murur

I have lost my passport : Waddart jawaaz safari : **(lost)**; dhayi, mafqud

I am from ... : Ana min ...

Seaport

Sea shore : Sahil-el-bahr

Sea sickness : Dokha

Seaport : Meenaa

Sea man : Mellah, pl. malalih

Ship : Baa-khira (or) Safeena, **(steamship)**; markab, pl. marakib

Boat : Qaareh (or) Filooka, safina, pl. safayin

Ticket : Attath-kira

Launch : Laanshya (or) Zaurekbukhari, markabsa ghir;

lanch

Goods : Bathaa-ya

Clearance : Tass-reeh

Export : Tas-deer, baath, yabath

Import : Tas-reed, dakhilat, waridat

Documents : Mus-tanadaat, wathiqa, pl. wathayiq

Parcels : Turood (pl) Tared(s)

Customs duties : Rusoom al-ghum-regh

Tax free : ma-fee min addareeba

Warehouse : Al-makh-zan

Paid : Mad-fooa(f) Mad-foo (m), mufi
In cash : Naq-dan
I have completed the necessary procedures :
Amalt al-ij-raa-at allazima
Israel Boycott office : Mak-tab muqata-at israaeel

Not on the black-list : Mush-fee al-qaayemaassauda

Post Office
(Maktal al-bareed)

Mail : Posta, V. baath-y, bath

Postman : Saaee-bareed, bustajee, postachi

Post master : Mudir-posta

Post Box : Sandoogh al-bareed

Express Letter : Rissalah-kusta-jila

Letter : Jawaab, pl. jawabaat, maktoob

Registered Letter : Mutaahad

Stamp (postage) : Taabaa, pl. tawaabaa; bareed

Money order : Hawaalah-bareed yyah

Parcel : Qit-aa, amana, pl. amayin

Envelope : Jarfi gawab, tharaf(s),thuroof (pl.)

Air mail : Bareed jawwe, bareed aelgaewwi

Telegram : Teleghraf, ol. teleghraft, barqiyeh

Address : Enwaan

Telephone Haatif, V. haka BI telfon;
(call) mukaalmah, pl.mukaalmaat
Wireless : Haatif, tel

BANK : Bunk, pl. bunuk, mas-raf

Cheque : Hawala, pl. hawayil, sack/ shaik(s), shaikaat (pl.)

Travelling cheque : Shaik-seeyaache

Cash : Nuqud

Salary : Raatib, maash, pl. maasht,**(money)**; flus, fulus

Hospital
(musteshfa, pl. musteshayat) Pharmacy

Where is the nearest pharmacy/chemist? :
Wain ag-rab saidaliya?

What time does it open? : Saa-a kam taf-tah?

I need some medicines: Nebbi baa-th al-ad-wiya

Here is the prescription : Hathi-he was-fat attabeeb

Is there a doctor? : Andakum ductoor? (or)Tabeeb

Yes, there is one in this street :
Ay-wa fee waahad fee hatha ashaara

Call an ambulance : Naadi sayarat al-is-aaf

I have a pain here : Andi waja (or) Alam hana

Please Note :
Various Body Organs Chapter : 4 Page 12

Shopping

How much is this? : Bikam hada? (or) Hatha?;
(cost) : Qima, pl. aqyam

Is this for Sale? : Hal-hatha lel-bea? **(Sale)**; bi
(For sale); lilbi

It is : Ay-wa.

No, it is not. : La, mush lel-bea.

How much a kilo? : Baish el-kilo?

How much a litre? : Baish-el-litra?

Expensive, dear : Ghaali

Cheap, low price : Rakhees (or) Mush-ghaali

The shop : Addukan (or) Al-matjar

The customer : Azzuboon (m), **(customer)**;
mustehlik Azuboona (f)

I want half a kilo of... : Enreed nasf kilo min...

Quarter of... : Enreed ruba kilo min...

Give me : Ateeni

Send this to... : Ersil hatha ila..., baath, yibath

Change (alter) this : Ghayyer hatha, Tabdil, khurda

Change (exchange) : Sarref

CHAPTER—II

Useful Grammar
Grammar : Nahuwa Sarf

Pronouns		Possessive	Arabic Suffixes
I	Annaa	My book Kita**bi**	I (or) ee
We	Nahnu	Our book Kitaab**na**	na Neh-Na
He	Huwa	His book Kitaab**ah**	Ah(or) hu
She	Heya	Her book Kitaab**ha**	ha
IT	Huwa	(or) Heya Its	Ah(or)hu
They	Henn (f)	Their book Kitaab**henn**	Henn
They	Hum (m)	Their book Kitaab**hum**	Hum
You	Enta (m) s, Enta,	Your book Kitaab**ak**	Ak
You	Anti (f) s. Enti,	Your book Kitaab**ik**	Ik
You	Antum (m) pl, Entum	Your book Kitaab**kum**	Kum
You	Anten (f) pl, Entan	Your book Kitaab**ken**	Ken

Objective Pronouns

		Call = (Naandi)
Me -	Call Me	Naadi **Ni**
Us -	Call Us	Naadi **Na**
Him -	Call Him	Nadi **H**
Her -	Call Her	Naadi
Ha		
Them - (f)	Call Them	Naadi
Hen		
Them - (m)	Call Them	Naadi
Hum		
You - (m) s. (Onaadi)	I Call you	Naadi **Ka**
You - (f) s.	I Call You	Naadi **Ki**
You - (m) pl.	I Call You	Naadi
Kum		
You - (f) pl.	I Call you	Naadi **Ken**

Demonstratives

This - Hatha (m) (s) Hathi-hi (f) (s)

That - Hathak (m) (s) Hathik (f) (s)

These- Hathom (m) (pl.) Hathein (f) (Pl)

Those- Hathok (m) (pl.) Hathikahen (f) (Pl.)

Relative Pronouns

Who-whom-that Llli

When (time) Kaif (or) endama

Where (place) Llli... fee (or) haithu

While (time) Lamma

How Kaif

Who...? Man...?

Whom...? Man...?

Whose...? Lee-man (or) emta'man?

Which...? Ay-en...?

What...? Maatha

Where...? Wain...? (or) menain...?

Why...? Laysh...? (or) leemaatha...?

How...? Kaif...?

How many...? Kam (or) gheddash....?

How much...? Beish (or) bekam...?

How long...? Kam...?

How far...? etc. Kam

Nouns and Adjectives

Nouns and adjectives can be made feminine by suffixing the letter (a) for the singular and (at) for the plural.

Comparisons

More than	Ak-thar min
Less than	Aqal min
Good	Hasan
Better	Ah-san
Bad	Radee
Worse	Radee
The best	Al-ah-san
The worst	Al-ar-da

Adverbs

Always	Day-man
Badly	Ala nah-oo radee
By chance	Be-assod-fa
For the time being	Fee al-wagt al-haadar
Only	Bass or Faqat
Openly	Be-saraaha
Quietly	Be-hudoo
Seldom	Naa-diran
Sometimes	Ah-yaanan
Usually	Adatan
Well	Hassan

Interrogatives

Interrogative sentences are generally made by either a tone of voice of the word Hall as a prefix. e.g.

Do you know the way? Ta-ref attareegh? or
Hal-ta-ref attareegh?

Have you a pencil? Andak galam?
Hal-andak galam?

Prepositions

	Arabic	Example
(1) **By, with**	Be	By car besa yarrah with pen: Bel kalam.
(2) **For**	Le	For school: Le madrasa
(3) **For you**	Lak	
(4) **In**	Fee	In the House: Fee-al-
bayt		
(5) **From**	Min	From India: Min alhind
(6) **Because**	Le,	Anna Happy Because: Anna masroor
(7) **O**	Yaa	O My lord: Yaa rabee

Plurals

The suffix (In) is for all male Regular Nouns

The suffix (At) is for all Female Regular Nouns

A Teacher (m) Mudarris	Teachers
	Mudarris (In)
A Woman Teacher (f)	Women Teachers
Mudarrisa	Mudarris (At)

Irregular nouns are formed by an internal change and they must be memorised e.g.

Pen (s)	Galam (s) Ag-lam (pl)
Window (s)	Shubbak
Man (s) men	Rajel (s) Rajaala (pl)
Monkey (s)	Gherd (s) Ghorood (pl)
Door (s)	Baab (s) Be-baan (pl)

N.B. The Particle (EIN) is placed after a noun to mean duality eg.

A book	Kitaab
Two books	Kitabe**in**

Verb (Present Tense)

I am	Ana
You are	Anta (m) Anti (f)
He is	Huwa
She is	Heya
It is	Huwa (m) Heya (f)
We are	Nah-nu
They are	Hum (m) Henna (f)

Verb (Past Tense)

I was	Kunt
You were	Kunt (s) kuntum (pl)
He	Kan
She was	Kanat
It	Kan (m) kanan (f)

N.B. The Verb to Be in the Present Tense is rarely used in Conversation.

Verb To Have

I have	Andi
You have-singular	Andak (m) Andik (f)
You have-plural	Andakum (m) Andaken (f)
He has	Andahu
She has	Andaha
We have	Andaha
They have	Andahum (m) Andahen (f)
I had	Kan andi
You had	Kan andak (m) Kan andik (f)
We had	Kan andana
They had	Kan andahum (m) Kan andahen (f)
She had	Kan andaha
He had	Kan andahu

Useful Verbs

	Past Tense	Present	Command
To arrive	Wasal	Yasell	-
To ask	Sa-al	Yes -al	Is-al
To bring	Jaab	Yijeeb	Jeeb
Can	Gh-dar	Yagh-dar	-
To call	Naada	Yenaadi	Naadi
To carry	Hamal	Yeh-mal	Ih-mal
To carry	Shaal	Yesheel	Sheel
To change	Baddala	Yebaddel	Baddil
To clean	Naddafa	Yenaddaf	Naddif
To come	Jaa	Eejee	Ta-aal
To cook	Tabbakha	Yatabbakh	At-bekh
To drive	Saagh	Yisoogh	Soogh
To explain	Fahama	Yef-ham	If-ham
To forget	Nasa	Yansa	Ansa
To give	Ata	Ya-tee	A-tee
To go	Masha	Yemshi	Imshi
To hear	Sammaa	Yas-maa	Is-maa

	Past Tense	Present	Command
To inform	Balagha	Yeballegh	Balligh
To know	Arafa	Ya-ref	A-ref
To learn	Ta-allam	Yata-allem	Ta-allem
To leave	Taraka	Yet-rek	At-rek
To like	Habba	Yi-hibb	Hibb
To lock	Sakkar	Yessaker	Sakker
To look for	Dawwar	Yeddawer	Dawwer
Must	- Yajib -		
To open	Fataha	Yaf-tah	Af-tah
To put	Hatta	Ye-hett	Hett
To read	Ghara	Yegh-ra	Agh-ra
To rest	Staraah	Yestareeh	Istareeh
To repair	Sallaha	Yasallah	Sallah
To ride	Rakiba	Yar-kib	Ar-Kib
To say	Ghaal	Yeghool	Ghool
To see	Shaaf	Yishoof	Shoof
To sell	Ba'ah	Yabee	Beea
To send	Arsala	Yer-sil	Ar-sil
To show	Warra	Yewarri	Warri
To shut	Qafala	Yaq-fil	Iq-fil

	Past Tense	Present	Command
To sit	Jalasa	Yaj-lis	Ij-lis
To smoke	Dakh-khan	Yedakh-khen	Dakh-Khin
To speak	Takallam	Yetakallam	Takallam
To stand	Waqafa	Ya-qif	Qif
To sweep	Kanasa	Yes-nis	Ik-nis
To take	Akhada	Yakhud	Khud
To teach	Allama	Ye-allam	Allim
To tell	Ghaal	Yeghool	Ghool
To think	Fakkara	Ye-fakker	Fakker
To throw	Ramaa	Yar-me	Ar-me
To try	Jaraba	Ye-jarab	Ja-reb
To use	As-tamala	Yestamel	Istamel
To walk	Masha	Yemshi	Imshi
To want	Araada	Yi-reed	-
To wash	Ghasal	Yegh-sel	Igh-sil
To wear	Labasa	Yal-bes	Al-bis
To Under-stand	Fahama	Yef-ham	If-ham

CHAPTER—III
Time (1)

What time is it? : Kam assa-a? Besh es saa?
Saa-a kam tawwa?**Please** :Min-Fath-Lak, min-fath-lik (f)

It is one o'clock : Assa-a waheda

Two : Et-nein

Three : T'laata

Four : Ar-baa

Five : Khamsa

Six : Sitta

Seven : Sab-aa

Eight : T'manya

Nine : T'ssa-aa

Ten : Ash-raa

Eleven : Eh-daash

Twelve : At-naash

Five past one : Wahed wa khamsa

Ten past one : Wahed wa ash-raa

Quarter past one : Wahed wa rooba

Half past one : Wahed wa nesf

Twenty to two : Et-nein illa esh-reen

Quarter to two : Et-mein illa rooba

Ten to two : Et-mein illa ash-raa

Five to two : Et-nein illa khamsa

O'clock : Es saa

Minute : Daqiqa, Pl. Daqaayeq

Watch : Saa, Pl. Saat

Clock : Saa malat hyit

Watch maker : Saachi, Pl. saachiya

Watch hand : Sqrab

The watch goes : Es saa timsmi

The watch has stopped : Es saa wagifa

He wound, Winds : Nasab, Yansab

Spring : Zambrak

Glass, crystal : Jama, Balura

I do come early : Enjee bak-ree

At least once : Alal-aqal marraa waahcda

Time (2)

Why are you late? : Leematha/caysh anta

You are always late : Enta daaeeman muta-akhir

No, Never : Laa, abadan,
(But some times) Wa-Laakin, amynln

Come early tomorrow : Ta-aal back-ri buk-raa **(or)**
Ghod'wa

I will try to come in time: Sa-uhaawel enjee fi-al
Waqht

If I can : Thaa/Ghderi

Do not come late : Mat-jish-muta-akhir

I want to see you : Enreed enshoofak

Within : Khilaal (or) Dakhil

After : Ba-ad

You are one hour late : Enta lak sa-aa muta-akhir

It was cold last week : Kan fee bard fee al-usboo
al-maadi (or) Al-faayet

My watch is slow : Saa-ati muta-akhira

Your watch is fast : Saa-atak muta-qaddima

What time is it, Exactly now : Saa-kam?

Sometimes : Ah-yaanan (or) Baad-alwaqt, badhwaqt

At least once : Alal-Iaqal marraa

At once : Ferd Marra

As soon as, All at once : Haalama, Hessa, Halan

I finish my work : Entahee min shugh-lee

One by one : Wahid wahid **(Not one),**
La wahid, **(every one);** kull wahid

Help yourself : Ta-fadal (or) Tafathal

From ... to ... : Min ... ila ...

At four o'clock : Anda assaa-a ar-baa

late News : Akhbar Akhira

It is too late : Fat el waqt

Lately : Akhiran

Early : Min waqt, **(sooner);** qabl,
(soon); bil ajel, bissaa halan

Timely : Fi waqtuh

Leisure : Faragha

In the mean time : Fi dhak el/thna

By the time : Ala ma

For a time : La mudda

It is Late : Fayit waqt

For the time being : Fi hadhir

For a long time : Min zaman

In the course of time : Ma murur ez zaman

As soon as : Halan **(immediate)** saree, besur-a
(as soon as possible); fi awwal waqt

Time (3)

Today is a holiday : Al-youm ot-laa

It is a fine day : Nahaar Kuwais

Tomorrow is not a holiday : Bu-kra mush at-laa

Yesterday was a good day : Ams kaan nahaar kuwais

The day before yesterday : Awel-ams

... I was in : Ana-kunt fee

After tomorrow : Ba-ad buk-ra

I shall see you : En-shoofak (m)

Every other day : Youm ba-ad youm

Every day : Kul-youm, Pl. Ayam (days)

Today : Ae-youm

Daily : Yomi, Pl. Yomian, **(Opposite Night)** Jahar

Every week : Kul (every)es-boo, usbv, Pl. asabi, sabaya **(week)**

Weekly : Usbuii

Every month : Kul-sha-har,**(Months)**: Pl. Ishhur

Monthly : Shahri, Pl. Shahriyan

Two weeks : Es-boo-ain **(a fort night)**

Every Year : Kul-sana, Pl. Sanawat, senin,
(Last year), Elam,**Year Before Last** : awwal elam

Yearly : Senawi

Morning : Sabaah, Subh

Noon : Dhu-hr, Thuher (or) Nesfnahaar

M'd day-midnight : dhahm, Nesf-nahaar-Nesfallail

Before noon : Gabl athuher

Afternoon : Ba-ad athu-her

Night : Layl, Lail, Lela, Plilyayali, **(tonight)**; Hellela, **(By Night)**; Bil Lel

Day & Night : Lel wa nahar

Always : Day-man, Kull waqt

Early in the morning : Bad-ri fee assabaah

Late : Muta-akhir **(deceased)**; Marhum

Never : Abadan

Now : Al-aan (or) Tawa

Week Days
Friday : Al-jum-aa, Yom el juma

Saturday : As-sabt, Yom es sebt,

saturday night: Lelat el ahad

Sunday : Al-a-had, Yom elahad,

sunday evening: Mesa el ahad

Monday : Al-et-nain, yom el thnen,el/thnen

Tuesday : At-talaat, Yom eth thalatha

Wednesday : Al-erbiha, Yom el Arbaa

Thursday : Al-khamees, Yomelkhamis

Months of The Year
January : Yennayer, Kanun Thani

February : Feb-rayer, Shabat

March : Maars, Adhar

April : Ab-reel, Nisan

May : Maayou, Ayar

June : Youniyou, Haziran

July : Youliyou, Tamuz

August : Aghusts, Ad

September : Seb-tember, Elul

October : Ok-toober, Tishrin Awwal

November : Noovember, Tishrin Thani

December : Deecember, Kanun Awwal

What is the date to day? : Shinu attarikh al-youm?

What month : Ai sha-harr? (or) Fe-aysha-harr?

It is June (etc). : Sha-harr youniyou?

We are having a party next month :
Andana haf-la asha-har ajjaee.

The Colours

Colour (s) : Loan (s) al-waan (pl)

White : Baitha (f) Ab-yath(m),Beethcm, Pl.), Bedha Bayadh

Black : Sawda (f), As-wad (m), Sood(m, Pl.)

Green : Akh-dar (or) Akh-thar (f) Khadhra

Red : Ah-marr (m), Hamra (f), Humr.

Yellow : (m) As-far, (f) Safra, Pl.Sufr

Brown : (m) Esmer, As-mar(f) Samr, Pl. Sumur.

Gray : (m) Ra-maadi, Eshheb (f) Zimaadia

Blue : (m) Az-ragh, Ajraq,(f) Zarga, Zirqa, (Pl.) Zirq.

Zurugh

Violet : Banaf-saji, Benefsha, Benefshi

The Cardinal Points (Direction: Tarf)

East : Sharq, Eastward: sharqan
West : Gharb, Gharbi
North : Shamaal, bahri
South : Jenoob, kibli

Weathers

Weather, Climate : Taqs, Hawaa, Manaakh

Good Weather : Jameel, Dry

Climate : Manaakh, Jaff

Cold : Baard, Barid,Pl.Bardanin,Baridin

Hot : Pl Haamee,Harrin, Haar

Air-Wind : Hawaa-Reeh

Sky-Rain : Sema, Samma Matar, Matr, Tamtarck

Warm : Daff, Daffi, Sa Akhen

Sweat : Ya-Ragh, Yaraq, Araq, Arq

Shade - Clear : Thill, Fe-Saafi, Saffa, Dhahir, Vadhih

It is dusty today : Ajaaj al-youm

It is cold today : Bard al-youm

It is hot : Haarr (hamoo) (colloq.)

It is windy : Reeh-waajid (colloq.)

It is rainy : Fee-matar al-youm

It is very cold : Bar-d shadeed

Human Relations

Mother Country : El-Watn El-Asali

Person : Shakhs, Pl. Ashkhas

Person (I) : Mutekellim

Person (II) : Mukhata

Person (III) : Shakhs, Pl. Ashkas, Ghayib

Father : Al-abb, Abe, Pl. Aba, Abahat, Walid

Mother : Al-umm, Umm, Pl. Ummahat, Walida

Boy : Ibin, Al-walad, Walad, Pl. Awlad. Sabai, Pl. Sabyan

Girl : Ib-Nah, Al-Bint, Bint, Pl. Banat, Buneya, Pl.Buneyat

Children : Al-aw-laad, Awlad

Child : Al-walad, walad

Brother : Al-akh, Akh, Pl. Ikhwa, Ikhwan

Sister : Al-ukh-t, ukmt, Pl. Khawat

Daughter (s) : Bint, Al-bint (s) –Banaat (pl), Ib-nah

Husband : Zauj, Zaw-j, Zoji, Pl. Ajwaj, Rijul, Pl. Rijal
Rihal, Pl. Rwajil

Wife : Zawa, Zaw-ja, Zoja, Pl.
Zojat, Madam, Pl. Madamat
Sweetheart : Habeeba (f), Habeebcm
Lady (ladies) : Sitt (s) - Sittaat (pl),Khatun, Pl. Khawatin

Uncle (paternal) : Am, Al-amm, Pl. Amam
Aunt (paternal) : Al-ammah, Amma, Pl.Ammat
Uncle (maternal) : Khaal, Pl. Akhwal, Khawal
Aunt (maternal) : Khaala, Pl. Khalat

Brother-in-law : Nasib
Father-in-law : Al-amm, Hammu, Amm (Moslem)
Son-in-law : Zoj Bint, Khatn
Mother -in-law : Al-ammah, Hamat

Niece : Ib-net al-akh (m), Bintelakh (m) Ib-net al-ukht (f)
Bint-El-Ukht (f)

Nephew : Iben-al-akh (m) Iben-al-ukh-t (f)

Grandmother : Jaddta Jadda, Jidda, Pl.Jiddat

Grandfather : Jadd, Jidd, Pl. Ajdad

Grandchild : Hafid, Pl. Hafada

Cousin : Ibin-am (m), Bint-am (m), Ibin-Amma (f)

Fiance, Fiancee : Khateeb, Khateeba

Bride Groom : Arees, Aris

Bride : Aroosa, Arus

Wedding : Urss, Zafaaf, Nikah, Zawaj, Barrakh

Widow : Armala, Pl. Aramil, Qaabilah-midwife

Widower : Armal, Maratuh, Meyyita

Divorce : Talaagh, Talaaq, Yutalliq

Relation : Qarib, Pl. Qarayib,Qaraaba

Related to : Yakhuss

Family : Ayela, Pl. Avelat, Ayal, Us-Ra

Tribe : Ashira, Pl. Ashayir

Friend (m) : Sadeeq. Pl. asdiqaa
Friend (f) : Sadeeqa, Pl. saadiqaat

"Arabic Language Learning
By Medical & Paramedical Staff"
'Supplement: Common Use Arabic'.

"ABOUT THE AUTHOR"

"CURRICULUM-VITAE"

PROF.(DR.) ANIL K. SAHNI   Address: A-1/F-1 Block-A Dilshad Garden
B.Sc, M.B.B.S, M.S, F.I.C.S. Advanced D.H.A   Delhi-110095 India.
SURGEON, UROLOGIST, ENDOSCOPIST,
LITHOTRIPSY SPECIALIST.
LIFE MEMBER :   Mobile 09873083100
AUSTRIAN MEDICAL SOCIETY   E-mail dranil_sahni@yahoo.co.in
THE ASSOCIATION OF SURGEONS OF INDIA   dranil_sahni@hotmail.com
DELHI UROLOGICAL SOCIETY   dranilksahni@gmail.com
ASSOCIATION OF MINIMAL ACCESS SURGEONS OF INDIA
INDIAN ASSOCIATION OF GASTRO-INTESTINAL ENDOSURGEONS
MEDICAL COUNCIL OF INDIA REG.No.: 3599(06.01.2005) / 27417(30.05.1983)U.P.
DATE OF BIRTH : 02-06-1958
"QUALIFICATIONS": PASSED ALL EXAMS IN FIRST ATTEMPT WITH POSITION.
B.Sc :1977, Rohilkhand University, Bareilly. Merit Position, National Scholarship
M.B.B.S :1983, G.S.V.M. Medical College, Kanpur.
M.S : 1986, G.S.V.M. Medical College, Kanpur.
F.I.C.S 1995-96, International College of Surgeons, Chicago, Illinois, USA.
ADHA (Advanced Diploma Hospital Administration) : 2006, Institute of Health Care Administration,Chennai.
"EXTRA CURRICULUM":First Aid Certificate,1968, NSS & NCC Certification,1975-77,
Joint Treasurer, Physiology Society,1978: Executive Member, Socio-Cultural Society, G.S.V.M. Medical College,
Kanpur, 1982 Etc., Sports, Music, Print - Live Media & Others.
"EXPERIENCES"   (A)TEACHING EXPERIENCE:
DEMO./TUTOR/REG./RSO/SR:-GSVM Med.Coll.Kanpur (31.05.83 To 31.08.86);3 Yrs & 3 Months
    -MCKR Hosp.& Ayur.Res.Inst.Delhi:(10.11.87 To 30.06.89); 1 Year & 8 Months
    -Yashoda Hospital,Ghaziabad..: (1.1.1993 To 1.12.1994); 2 Years
ASSISTANT PROFESSOR (SURGERY) :- SantoshMed.Coll.Ghaziabad:(06.04.98 To 26.03.2001);2Yrs&11Months
    - SRMS IMS,Bareilly:(1.07.2004 To17.05.2006);1Yr & 11 Months
    - M.M.C.H., Muzaffarnagar: (18.05.06 To 31.08.07); 1Yr & 4 Months
    - M.A.M.C., Agroha (Hisar): (1.09.07 To 31.06.08); 10 Months
    ADDITIONAL :Urology,Lithotripsy,Non-Invasive/Minimal Invasive Surgery, Endoscopy,
    Surgical Teaching, BPT(Physio-Therapy) Courses, G.J Univ.Hisar.
ASSOCIATE PROFESSOR (SURGERY):-M.A.M.C.,Agroha(Hisar):(1.07.08 To 15.03.09);9Months
    -VCSG Govt.Med.Sciences & Res.Inst. Sri-Nagar,Pauri-Garhwal:
    [Offi.HOD, Act.MS, As Need],Co-ChairMan'CME','CPD'...,
    I/C Med.Edu.Unit; 15/16.03.2009 - Till Date.
PROFESSOR: Forwarded & Recommended Thrice, Confirmed(MCI)
    w.e.f 01/07/2011, Complete Experience & Publications Including Books.
(B) ASSOCIATED ASSIGNMENTS(TRAINING):Esteemed Tertiary Care Hospitals, P.G Teaching, DNB Courses:
    -Sir Ganga Ram Hospital, Delhi: (Dec. 1998 To Dec. 2001); About (3) Year
    -Narendra Mohan Hospital, Ghaziabad: (08.05.1999 To June 2005); About (6) Years
    -Surya Hospital, Delhi:About (4)Years & Others: In Various Capacities , Including "ADMINISTRATION".
(C) FOREIGN ASSIGNMENTS: -National Imnian Oil Company Hospitals,Iran. - About (1)One Year,
    17.12.1991 To 17.12.1992.
    -Aviation & Submarine (Metiga) Hospital, Tripoli, Libya. – About (1) One Year,
    26.05.1996 To 25/26. 05. 1997.
Versatile, Wide, Experience In Gen. Surgery, Urology , Lithotripsy & Working Experience Of Other
Surgical Super Specialties, Including Intensive Care (Incharge ICU).
"Advanced Diploma In Health Administration" & - Others : Certification In Process.
"(CME),(CPD),(LLL)...: Various National & InterNational Medical Education Programmes,Constant Participation
Throughout, Graduation Onwards,
About(>50) National & International Conferences, Seminars, Symposiums Etc. Participation By Important
'Scientific Studies', Useful Presentations, Discussions,Chairing Session, Publications.
-"3rd AMASI Skill Course", AIIMS, N.Delhi, 29th Nov. - 1st Dec.2006.
-"N.S.V Training Course": PGIMS, Rohtak, March'2008 ; C.S.M Medical University Lucknow, September'2011.
-"Post Graduate Surgical Course", Royal College Of Surgeons Of Edinburgh, U.K, Oct.'2008.
-"MCI CoOrdinatorsOrientationProgr.(1Day):MCIBasicWorkshop(3)Days,MCINodalCentreCMCLudhiana:Sept.2009.
-"AIIMS Ultrasound Trauma LifeSupport (AUTLS) Course",ASITECH,ASICON'2010, AIIMS,N.Delhi,15-20Dec.2010.
"About (50) : Publications, Including Books: **1."Arabic Language. . ."**RNI, I & B Ministry,GOI,2003,Several
Reprints, 'Supplement',Consideration By UN,ICRC,WHO & Others **2." Students Surgery Manual"**, Dec.2010...
"About (>25) 'Scientific Presentations': Computronics Media Publications,Colloborating Trauma,Filariasis,
Breast Care Global Projects ICMR & Others
*About (20): 'Scientific Projects'(In Process): Common Clinical Entities, Useful 'Research Projects' & Or
'Thesis Topics', Including Books. **"Surgery For Physio-Therapists" & "Essentials Of Litho-Tripsy".**
' Name, Selected, Nominated, Proposed, Published With Other Esteemed Personalities, Of Different
Pioneering Magnitudes, By Various National & InterNational Reputed Institutions.

www.ingramcontent.com/pod-product-compliance
Lightning Source LLC
Chambersburg PA
CBHW051721170526
45167CB00002B/746